LIBRARY

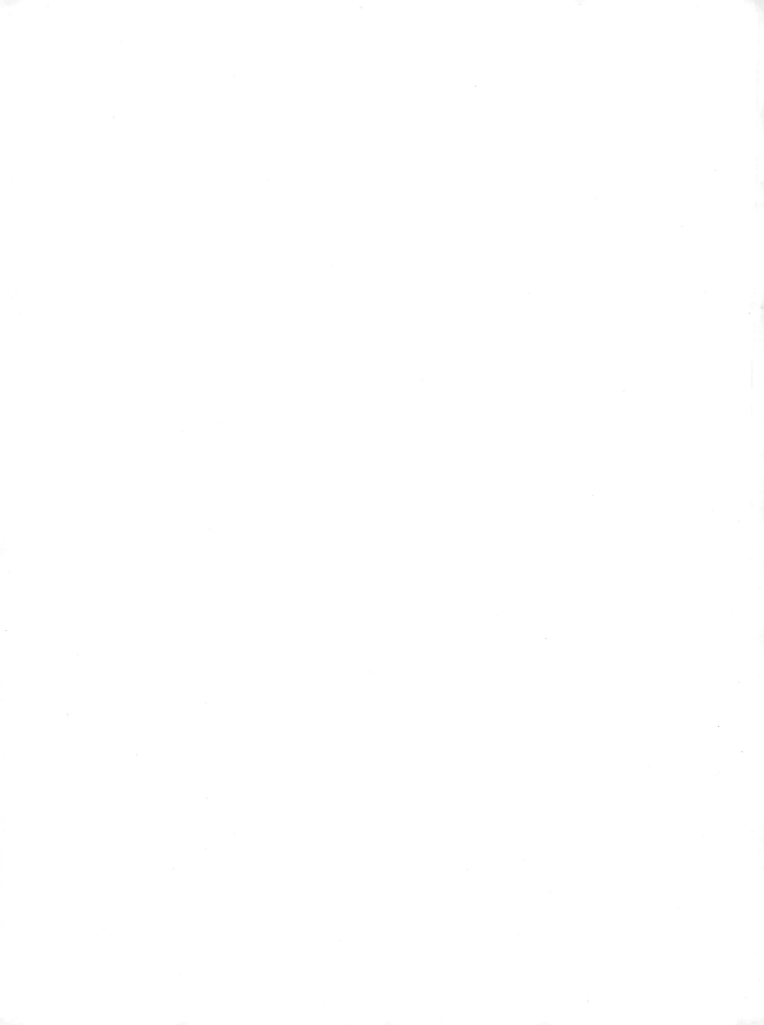

Chest Pain with Normal Coronary Arteries

Juan Carlos Kaski • Guy D. Eslick
C. Noel Bairey Merz

Editors

Chest Pain with Normal Coronary Arteries

A Multidisciplinary Approach

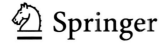 Springer

Editors

Juan Carlos Kaski, MD, DSc, FRCP,
FESC, FACC, FAHA
Division of Clinical Sciences
Cardiovascular Sciences Research Centre
St. George's University of London
Cranmer Terrace
London
UK

C. Noel Bairey Merz, MD, FACC, FAHA
Barbra Streisand Women's Heart Center
Cedars-Sinai Heart Institute
Los Angeles, California
USA

Guy D. Eslick, DrPH, PhD, FACE, FFPH
Department of Surgery
The Whiteley-Martin Research Centre
The University of Sydney, Sydney
Australia

ISBN 978-1-4471-4837-1   ISBN 978-1-4471-4838-8   (eBook)
DOI 10.1007/978-1-4471-4838-8
Springer London Heidelberg New York Dordrecht

Library of Congress Control Number: 2013934226

Printed on acid-free paper

Springer is part of Springer Science+Business Media (www.springer.com)

This book is dedicated to all researchers worldwide who over the years have contributed to the understanding of this puzzling condition. In particular, to those who dared thinking beyond the boundaries of established "dogma" and constituted an example for newer generations of physicians and scientists.

Foreword

I am honored and grateful to the authors of this timely volume *Chest Pain with Normal Coronary Arteries* for asking me to write a Foreword for it.

The volume covers, with 32 well integrated chapters, a topic which until now had received insufficient attention because it departs from a deeply established paradigm which I have witnessed over the past 50 years, and still largely conditions cardiac thinking, practice and research.

At medical school, in the 1950s, I was taught that the progression of atherosclerosis reduced coronary flow reserve until the development of coronary insufficiency resulted in effort angina and, when more severe, in acute, myocardial infarction. Thrombosis was by many considered a consequence rather than the cause of acute infarction. The Cardiology textbook by Friedberg stated that "angina might occur also at rest but, if it did not occur also on effort, had a non ischemic origin".

Thus angina could only be caused by an excessive myocardial demand in the presence of obstructive coronary atherosclerosis, and patients with acute infarction were prescribed strict bed rest for 3 weeks as their coronary flow reserve was thought to be exhausted! Accordingly drugs that increased myocardial blood flow in animals, such as dipyridamole, were developed and the beneficial effects of nitrates were attributed to a reduced myocardial demand, rather than to dilatation of constricted vessels.

The first challenge to this dogma came in 1959 from clinical observations by Prinzmetal suggesting that angina at rest with preserved effort tolerance (variant angina) could be caused by an increase in "tonus" at the site of a subcritical stenosis, resulting in transient occlusion.

Fourteen years later, spasm was also described at the site of non-stenosed arteries (the variant of the variant), yet also today, in many institutions spasm is suspected and searched for only in patients with severe symptoms but angiographically normal arteries! The presence of a stenosis by itself is thought a sufficiently plausible cause for angina on effort or at rest!

A second challenge came in the 1970s when the use of Holter recordings allowed the demonstration of ischemic episodes during daily life not preceded by an increased heart rate, the major determination of myocardial demand, suggestive of transient coronary vasoconstriction. Thus the concept of dynamic coronary stenosis became accepted. Subsequently, in 1990, a large variability in residual flow reserve was reported also in selected patients with an isolated single total coronary occlusion, preserved ventricular function and no other stenosis, suggesting that regional coronary flow could be modulated, not only by dynamic stenoses, but also by distal, small coronary vessels constriction.

Thus although overwhelming evidence indicates that coronary vasoconstriction can cause ischemia in the presence of coronary atherosclerosis, the notion that vasoconstriction of large and small coronary branches can cause ischemia and angina also in the absence of coronary stenoses is still not sufficiently prevalent in some catheterization laboratories, as when no stenoses are found the patient's anginal symptoms are often labeled as "non-cardiac"!

This volume is very timely and will most likely serve the important purpose of stimulating clinical investigators with inquisitive minds to dare focusing their research interests on the yet unknown multiple aspects of coronary blood flow regulation and mechanisms of myocardial ischemia, identification of clinical patient subsets, and the varied potential pathogenic mechanisms responsible for myocardial ischemia in patients with angiographically normal coronary arteries. For this challenge, the 32 chapters that compose the book are all pieces of a clever jigsaw puzzle.

In this innovative task I hope for investigators to be "splitters" rather than "lumpers" and to make an effort to discover relevant associations that link specific pathogenic mechanisms with distinctive clinical symptoms and specific instrumental descriptors rather than searching for single common denominators. In this way, only, the treatment of chest pain can become personalized – patient oriented – rather than standardized and disease oriented.

Prof. Attilio Maseri

Preface

The condition known as "chest pain with normal coronary arteries" or "cardiac syndrome X" has, practically since the advent of coronary arteriography, puzzled physicians and patients alike. Although epicardial coronary artery spasm, as seen in Prinzmetal's variant angina, explains a proportion of cases of typical chest pain despite normal coronary arteriograms, many patients who seek medical attention for exertional and rest angina in the absence of obstructive coronary artery disease are not variant angina cases. The syndrome thus continues to represent a "mystery", rather than a reality, for many in clinical practice. This monographic work, written by many of the most active research groups in the field in different continents, comprehensively tackles the clinical presentation and the pathogenesis of the condition, as well as its management. The syndrome constitutes both a diagnostic and therapeutic challenge.

Women represent a large proportion of the population affected by microvascular dysfunction, believed to be the main pathogenic mechanism of the syndrome, once extracardiac causes of chest pain and variant angina have been excluded. Several chapters in the book deal with aspects directly related to this issue. Contrary to epicardial coronary artery disease, abnormalities of the coronary microcirculation have remained elusive to conventional imaging techniques and only recently researchers appear to be making progress in obtaining much needed information in this field. The present monographic work addresses this aspect of the problem and proposes useful clinical diagnostic algorithms, thus bringing this subject closer to the practicing cardiologist. The functional aspects of the coronary microcirculation, its clinical presentation and prognosis, as well as the diagnostic tests used for the assessment of microvascular dysfunction are important topics highlighted in the book.

The syndrome of chest pain with angiographically normal coronary arteries is not a "rare" syndrome, as over 50 % of patients undergoing diagnostic angiography for the assessment of typical chest pain suggestive of coronary atherosclerosis is found not to have obstructive coronary artery disease. Epidemiological considerations, socio-economic issues, differential diagnoses and gender differences in diagnosis and management are all addressed in specific chapters in the book. Importantly, the condition can – and often does – impair the patient's quality of life and trigger serious psychological disturbances, as discussed in detail in the present monographic work. An adverse prognosis has been reported in certain patient subgroups, and this topic is also tackled in *ad hoc* chapters in the book. Although treatment remains problematic, management strategies are proposed in the book that can improve the patient's symptoms, quality of life and wellbeing. The present work also proposes new research needed to identify the different patient subgroups encompassed by this heterogeneous syndrome, understand its pathogenic mechanisms further and devise newer, more effective therapies. We hope that this book will be a useful practical tool for the clinician, a bank of information for those interested in understanding the causes and mechanisms of the condition and a source of inspiration for both scientists and clinical researchers who work in the field. The ultimate expectation, however, is that the present book helps us in managing our patients better.

Acknowledgments

We are grateful to the authors of the various chapters of this book who generously devoted time to make this monographic work a reality. We are also indebted to the multitude of patients who have, over the past decades, helped researchers carry out investigations to understand the condition better.

Contents

Contributors

Sami R. Achem, MD, FACP, FACG, AGAF Division of Gastroenterology, Mayo College of Medicine, Mayo Clinic Florida, Jacksonville, FL, USA

Cristina Almansa, MD, PhD Division of Gastroenterology, Mayo College of Medicine, Mayo Clinic Florida, Jacksonville, FL, USA

Giuseppe Ambrosio, MD, PhD Division of Cardiology, University of Perugia, Perugia, Italy

Tarek Francis Antonios, MBChB (Hons.), MSc, MD, FESC, FRCP Department of Clinical Science, St George's University of London, London, UK

Anastasios Athanasiadis, MD Department of Cardiology, Robert-Bosch-Krankenhaus, Stuttgart, Germany

C. Noel Bairey Merz, MD, FACC, FAHA Barbra Streisand Women's Heart Center, Cedars-Sinai Heart Institute, Los Angeles, CA, USA

John Beltrame, MBBS, PhD Discipline of Medicine, The Queen Elizabeth Hospital, University of Adelaide, Adelaide, SA, Australia

Raffaele Bugiardini, MD Department of Internal Medicine, Cardio-Angiology and Hepatology, University of Bologna, Bologna, Italy

Paolo G. Camici, MD, FACC, FESC, FAHA, FRCP Department of Cardiology, Vita-Salute University and San Raffaele Scientific Institute, Milan, Italy

Brian G. Choi, MD, MBA Department of Medicine, George Washington University, Washington, DC, USA

Peter Collins, MA, MD (Cantab), FRCP Clinical Cardiology and Physiology, NHLI, Imperial College London, and Royal Brompton and Harefield NHS Foundation Trust, London, UK

Filippo Crea, MD Department of Cardiovascular Sciences, Università Cattolica del Sacro Cuore, Rome, Italy

Domenico G. Della Rocca, MD Division of Cardiovascular Medicine, University of Florida, Gainesville, FL, USA

Ingrid E. Dumitriu, MD, PhD Division of Clinical Sciences, Cardiovascular Sciences Research Centre, St. George's University of London, London, UK

Perry Elliott, MD, MBBS Department of Inherited Cardiovascular Disease, University College Hospital London, London, UK

Guy D. Eslick, DrPH, PhD, FACE, FFPH Department of Surgery, The Whiteley-Martin Research Centre, The University of Sydney, Sydney, NSW, Australia

Wafia Eteiba, MD Department of Epidemiology, Graduate School of Public Health, University of Pittsburgh, Pittsburgh, PA, USA

Andreas J. Flammer, MD Division of Cardiovascular Diseases, Department of Internal Medicine, Mayo Clinic and College of Medicine, Rochester, MN, USA

Augusto Gallino, MD Ospedale Regionale di Bellinzona e Tre Valli, Bellinzona, Switzerland

Peter Ganz, MD Division of Cardiology, San Francisco General Hospital, San Francisco, CA, USA, Center of Excellence in Vascular Research, University of California – San Francisco, San Francisco, CA, USA

Bernard J. Gersh, MB, ChB, DPhil, FRCP Division of Cardiovascular Diseases, Department of Internal Medicine, Mayo Clinic and College of Medicine, Rochester, MN, USA

Guarini Giacinta, MD Cardiovascular Medicine Division, Cardio Thoracic and Vascular Department, University of Pisa, Pisa, Italy

C. Prakash Gyawali, MD, MRCP Division of Gastroenterology, Barnes-Jewish Hospital, Washington University School of Medicine, St. Louis, MO, USA

Ralph Kent Hermsmeyer, PhD Research and Development, Dimera Incorporated, Portland, OR, USA

Juan Carlos Kaski, MD, DM (Hons), DSc, FRCP, FESC, FACC, FAHA Division of Clinical Sciences, Cardiovascular Sciences Research Centre, St George's University of London, London, UK

Gaetano Antonio Lanza, MD Department of Cardiovascular Sciences, Università Cattolica del Sacro Cuore, Rome, Italy

Amir Lerman, MD Division of Cardiovascular Diseases, Department of Internal Medicine, Mayo Clinic and College of Medicine, Rochester, MN, USA

Jannet F. Lewis, MD Department of Medicine, George Washington University Medical Center, Washington, DC, USA

Mario Marzilli, MD Cardiovascular Medicine Division, Cardio Thoracic and Vascular Department, University of Pisa, Pisa, Italy

Puja K. Mehta, MD Barbra Streisand Women's Heart Center, Cedars-Sinai Heart Institute, Los Angeles, CA, USA

Peter Ong, MD Department of Cardiology, Robert-Bosch-Krankenhaus, Stuttgart, Germany

Vimal Patel, MRCP, MBBS, BSc Department of Inherited Cardiovascular Disease, University College Hospital London, London, UK

Carl J. Pepine, MD Division of Cardiovascular Medicine, University of Florida, Gainesville, FL, USA

Anita Phan, MD Division of Cardiology, Cedars-Sinai Heart Institute, Los Angeles, CA, USA

Ornella E. Rimoldi, MD, FACC, FAHA IBFM CNR, Segrate, Italy

Diane L. Rosenbaum, MA Department of Psychology, University of Missouri-St. Louis, One University Boulevard, St. Louis, MO, USA

Thomas Rutledge, PhD, ABPP Department of Psychiatry, VA San Diego Healthcare System, San Diego, CA, USA

Karin Schenck-Gustafsson, MD, PhD Department of Medicine, Cardiac Unit, Karolinska Institutet and Karolinska University Hospital, Solna, Stockholm, Sweden

Udo Sechtem, MD Department of Cardiology, Robert-Bosch-Krankenhaus, Stuttgart, Germany

Anisa Shaker, MD Division of Gastroenterology, Barnes-Jewish Hospital, Washington University School of Medicine, St. Louis, MO, USA

Leslee J. Shaw, PhD Professor of Medicine, Emory University School of Medicine, Emory Program in Cardiovascular Outcomes Research and Epidemiology, Atlanta, GA, USA

Hiroaki Shimokawa, MD, PhD Department of Cardiovascular Medicine, Tohoku University Graduate School of Medicine, Sendai, Japan

Chrisandra Shufelt, MD, MS Barbra Streisand Women's Heart Center, Cedars-Sinai Heart Institute, Los Angeles, CA, USA

Rosanna Tavella, PhD, BSc (Hons) Department of Medicine, The Queen Elizabeth Hospital, The University of Adelaide, Adelaide, SA, Australia

Theresa Lee Thompson, PhD Research and Development, Dimera Incorporated, Portland, OR, USA

Louise E.J. Thomson, MBChB, FRACP S. Mark Taper Foundation Imaging Center, Cedars-Sinai Medical Center, Los Angeles, CA, USA

Isabella Tritto, MD Division of Cardiology, University of Perugia, Perugia, Italy

Giuseppe Vassalli, MD Department of Cardiology, Fondazione Cardiocentro Ticino, Lugano, Switzerland

Pierre Vogt, MD Department of Cardiology, Centre Hospitalier Universitaire Vaudois (CHUV), Lausanne, Switzerland

Talya Waldman, MSN, WHNP, NCMP Barbra Streisand Women's Heart Center, Cedars-Sinai Heart Institute, Los Angeles, CA, USA

Carolyn M. Webb, PhD Clinical Cardiology and Physiology, NHLI, Imperial College London, and Royal Brompton and Harefield NHS Foundation Trust, London, UK

Kamila S. White, PhD Department of Psychology, University of Missouri-St. Louis, One University Boulevard, St. Louis, MO, USA

Satoshi Yasuda, MD, PhD Department of Cardiovascular Medicine, National Cerebral and Cardiovascular Center, Suita, Japan

Cinzia Zuchi, MD Division of Cardiology, University of Perugia, Perugia, Italy

Part I

Introductory Chapters

Cardiac Syndrome X: An Overview

Juan Carlos Kaski, C. Noel Bairey Merz,
and Guy D. Eslick

Abstract

Patients with cardiac syndrome X (CSX), defined as typical chest pain associated with electrocardiographic changes suggestive of transient myocardial ischemia despite normal coronary angiograms, continue to constitute a diagnostic and a therapeutic challenge. CSX is not a "rare" syndrome, as up to 50 % of patients undergoing diagnostic angiography for the assessment of typical chest pain are found not to have obstructive coronary artery disease. CSX encompasses a variety of pathogenic subgroups and is most typically seen in peri- and postmenopausal women. The condition can impair the patient's quality of life, is associated with an adverse prognosis in certain patient subgroups, and represents a substantial cost burden to the healthcare system. Not infrequently, a lack of understanding of the pathogenesis of the syndrome by the treating physician results in poor management of the condition. Treatment remains elusive, but management strategies exist that can improve the patient's quality of life and wellbeing. Clinical trials are needed to evaluate the impact of management strategies on major adverse cardiac events. The present book addresses most of the important issues relevant to the understanding of the condition including its epidemiology, pathogenesis, diagnosis and effective management strategies.

Keywords

Cardiac syndrome X • Microvascular angina • Angina with normal coronaries • Pathophysiology

J.C. Kaski, MD, DM (Hons), DSc, FRCP, FESC, FACC, FAHA (✉)
Division of Clinical Sciences,
Cardiovascular Sciences Research Centre,
St George's University of London, Cranmer Terrace,
London SW17 0RE, UK
e-mail: jkaski@sgul.ac.uk

C.N. Bairey Merz, MD, FACC, FAHA
Barbra Streisand Women's Heart Center,
Cedars-Sinai Heart Institute, 444 S. San Vicente Blvd Suite 600,
Los Angeles, CA 90048, USA
e-mail: noel.baireymerz@cshs.org; merz@cshs.org

G.D. Eslick, DrPH, PhD, FACE, FFPH
Department of Surgery,
The Whiteley-Martin Research Centre,
The University of Sydney,
Sydney, NSW 2006, Australia
e-mail: guy.eslick@sydney.edu.au

Introduction

Although patients with typical exertional chest pain and positive exercise stress test results usually have obstructive coronary artery disease, particularly when conventional risk factors such as diabetes mellitus, hypertension, smoking and dyslipidemia are present, recent reports indicate that up to 50 % of these patients have no obstructive coronary artery disease [1]. Issues related to the incidence and epidemiology of CSX will be discussed by Tavella and Eslick in Chap. 4. Patients with systemic hypertension, left ventricular hypertrophy, cardiomyopathies and diabetes mellitus are often excluded from CSX series, as it is assumed that the cause for their angina is "known". However little justification exists for these exclusions, as the pathogenic mechanisms operating in these patients do not differ substantially from those in other CSX patients unaffected by those risk factors or co-morbidities. These issues are discussed by Lanza and Crea in Chap. 7 in the book. Patients with Prinzmetal's variant angina due to epicardial coronary artery spasm and those with objectively documented extra-cardiac causes for the pain such as the chest wall syndrome, psychological disturbances, and esophageal abnormalities need to be identified and treated accordingly, as suggested by Kaski et al. and Almansa and Achem in Chaps. 1 and 2, respectively.

Despite research efforts by different investigators on both sides of the Atlantic and Pacific in the past four decades, many questions remain regarding the pathogenesis of CSX. The intriguing relationship between CSX and pain perception abnormalities as well as the different mechanisms playing differing roles in subsets of patients encompassed by the syndrome of angina despite angiographicaly normal coronary arteries continue to represent research targets.

Pathogenesis

The pathogenesis of the condition will be discussed in detail in Chap. 7. Briefly, however, microvascular coronary dysfunction (MCD), expressed as either reduced coronary microvascular dilatory responses and/or increased coronary microvascular resistance or microvascular spasm, have been consistently reported in CSX patients. The named "microvascular angina" coined by Cannon in the 1980s [2] refers to this commonly found pathogenic mechanism. MCD has been shown to be responsible for regional myocardial blood flow abnormalities and heterogeneous myocardial perfusion [2–4].

New techniques for the assessment of MCD are discussed by Beltrame in Chap. 24 and the important of assessing abnormal vasomotion in the catheterization laboratory to characterize pathogenic mechanisms is presented by Ong et al. in Chap. 23. Endothelial dysfunction, with reduced bioavailability of endogenous NO and increased plasma levels of endothelin-1 (ET-1), may explain the abnormal behavior of the coronary microvasculature in CSX [4–6]. Transient myocardial perfusion defects have been reported in areas supplied by arteries showing endothelial dysfunction [4] and increased levels of ET-1 correlated, in several studies, with impaired coronary microvascular dilator responses in patients with chest pain and normal coronary arteries [7, 8]. Endothelial dysfunction in microvascular angina appears to be associated with several mechanisms, including the presence of conventional risk factors such as smoking, obesity, hypercholesterolemia, hypertension and inflammation [1]. High plasma C-reactive protein, a marker of inflammation, has been shown to correlate with disease activity [9] and endothelial dysfunction [4–8]. The presence of subangiographic coronary atheroma, not uncommonly present in individuals with microvascular angina, can impair endothelial function, as reported in Chap. 8 by Della Rocca and Pepine.

Insulin resistance has also been suggested to have a major pathogenic role in this condition; this issue is exhaustively discussed by Tritto et al. in Chap. 13. The high prevalence (approximately 70 % in most series) of postmenopausal women in the CSX population, has suggested a role for estrogen deficiency as a pathogenic mechanism [10]. As discussed in Chap. 29 by Shufelt and Waldman, estrogen deficiency acting via endothelium-dependent and endothelium-independent mechanisms can lead to microvascular angina [10]. Increased pain sensitivity has been also linked to estrogen deficiency in CSX [10]. Several studies have shown that Impaired endothelial function in postmenopausal CSX patients is improved by the administration of 17β-estradiol [10]. Chapters 30 and 32 by Hermsmeyer et al. and Bairey Merz et al., respectively, address important issues related to hormonal abnormalities other than estrogen deficiency as a potential mechanism for microvascular dysfunction in CSX.

Myocardial Ischemia

The development of transient ECG changes suggestive of myocardial ischemia is a requisite for the diagnosis of CSX. However, objective documentation of myocardial ischemia by means other than ST segment changes during pain has been reported in approximately 40 % of patients with chest pain and normal coronary angiograms. Thus, myocardial ischemia as objectively documented by perfusion scans, stress echocardiography or measurements of lactate in the coronary sinus, for example, has proven elusive in the majority of patients. More recently, however, studies using myocardial-perfusion magnetic resonance imaging (MRI) [11] and 31-Phosphorus nuclear MR [12] have provided evidence for myocardial ischemia in patients with chest pain and normal coronary arteries, as described by Thomson in Chap. 21. The roles of echocardiography and positron emission tomography in the diagnosis of CSX and the understanding of its underlying pathogenesis, is also tackled in the book by Lewis and Choi, and Camici and Rimoldi (Chaps. 22 and 20 respectively). Non-ischemic mechanisms have been proposed to explain the occurrence of ischemia-like ST segment changes in CSX, including autonomic nervous system dysfunction [13–15].

Abnormal Pain Perception

Increased pain perception is common in patients with CSX, but the reason for this remains elusive. Potassium and adenosine release, as well as abnormalities in the central modulation of pain perception, have been suggested to play a role [14, 15]. Greater and more extensive cortical activation, particularly of the right insula, suggesting abnormal handling of afferent stimuli by the central nervous system is seen in CSX patients as compared with controls [15]. CSX patients may thus have an ineffective thalamic gate that would allow inadequate cortical activation by afferent stimuli from the heart, resulting in increased pain perception [15]. Autonomic nervous system imbalance with increased adrenergic activity and impaired parasympathetic tone could explain both increased pain sensitivity and endothelial dysfunction [13–15]. Possible interactions between pain threshold and microvascular dysfunction in CSX have been proposed to explain the relatively common finding of severe chest pain in the absence of documentable myocardial ischemia [8]. Not as yet well defined interactions between chest pain and coronary microvascular dysfunction are likely to be important in the pathogenesis of CSX and may influence the patient's clinical presentation. It is conceivable that a given CSX patient with a markedly increased pain sensitivity (low threshold for pain) could develop chest pain in response to cardiac (and non-cardiac) stimuli able to activate pain receptors in the heart, even in the absence of major coronary microvascular dysfunction or the occurrence of myocardial ischemia [8]. Adenosine and potassium release have been suggested to cause chest pain and ECG changes in CSX patients even when myocardial ischemia is not present. Endothelin-1, estrogen levels and the autonomic nervous system modulate pain threshold. Patients with both a marked MCD leading to myocardial ischemia and a reduced pain threshold will most likely be highly symptomatic [8]. Patients with intermediate degrees of chest pain sensitivity and some MCD may have no detectable myocardial ischemia and symptoms can be of low or moderate intensity. Both pain threshold and MCD have ample gradation spectra regarding severity and are also modulated by factors such as endothelial dysfunction, hormonal influences, inflammation, the autonomic nervous system and psychological mechanism [8].

Thus variable interactions between pain threshold and MCD can explain the heterogeneous clinical presentation of CSX and the variable rates of myocardial ischemia in different research studies. Chapter 32 by Bairey Merz et al. addresses issues related to pain sensitivity and pain management in CSX.

Psychological Morbidity

Patients with chest pain despite normal coronary arteriograms have high rates of psychiatric morbidity [16]; approximately 30 % have a treatable psychiatric disorder and another 30 % have some psychological disorder. However, psychiatric morbidity varies in different series and may, particularly in patients with anxiety disorders, be secondary to inappropriate reassurance regarding the etiology and mechanisms of CSX and the cardiovascular symptoms that lead to an impaired quality of life. Patient uncertainties as to the prognosis of the condition may contribute to psychological morbidity. In Chap. 6, White and Rosenbaum exhaustively deal with these issues.

Cost Economics Issues

L Shaw, in Chap. 5, examines the data on costs of cardiovascular care for women and highlights the importance of chest pain and the burden of persistent angina as driving higher costs of care. A consistent body of evidence reports that women generally utilize more healthcare resources than men. A large component of the costs of care includes those for ongoing symptoms including the burden of angina. In the NIH-NHLBI Women's Ischemia Syndrome Evaluation (WISE) study, costs of care were estimated for symptomatic women with and without obstructive coronary artery disease. Even women with none to mild non-obstructive coronary artery disease had predicted lifetime costs of cardiovascular care of approximately 750,000 dollars. Thus the economic burden of angina, even in the setting of nonobstructive CAD, is costly and can result in high lifetime costs of care. Proper understanding of the condition should result in a reduction of this financial burden.

Prognosis and Quality of Life

Classical forms of CSX, characterized by the triad of chest pain, abnormal stress testing and completely normal coronary arteries, have been reported to have a benign prognosis [3]. More recent data in larger populations with longer follow-up time periods appear to suggest a relatively higher risk for adverse cardiac events [17] such as heart failure and hospitalization in those subjects with myocardial ischemia associated to MCD [18] Patients presenting with left bundle branch block and subjects with MCD secondary to serious systemic diseases (such as amyloidosis or myeloma), have an impaired prognosis regarding left ventricular function and survival, respectively. Specifically, CSX related to MCD has an adverse prognosis and health care cost expenditure comparable to obstructive CAD in both stable angina and unstable acute coronary syndrome patient populations, according to data assessed and discussed by Bairey Merz in Chap. 25. Invasive assessment of coronary reactivity testing, including endothelial and non-endothelial dependent vasomotion provides potent prognostic information in subjects with normal and minimally diseased coronary arteries. Additional assessment by non-invasively determined coronary or myocardial blood flow reserve provides additive prognostic value to routine coronary angiography. MCD predicts a relatively greater proportion of heart failure events compared to myocardial infarction, suggesting potential links between MCD and heart failure with preserved systolic function, although longer term follow-up of ventricular function has not been performed. Bairey Merz and colleagues argue that the high prevalence of this condition, adverse prognosis in certain patient subgroups and substantial health care costs, particularly in women, coupled with the lack of evidence-base regarding treatment, makes intervention trials in CSX and microvascular angina a research priority area.

In Chap. 26, Rutledge assesses the effects of CSX on quality of life and stresses the fact that although often considered a problem outside of the scope of standard medical care, quality of life is indirectly the most important target of most patient-health care provider relation. Improving physical function, reducing symptom burden, improving endurance, managing pain, helping patients return to work, decreasing depression and anxiety, and increasing independence "are among the many dimensions of quality of life enhanced from care received in cardiology and primary care settings. Poor quality of life is a frequent concern among patients with chest pain and normal coronary arteries or no obstructive coronary artery disease (CAD), with evidence that this population may endure greater quality of life impairment relative even to those with chest pain and obstructive CAD."

Management

The management of CSX is challenging and often frustrating for both patient and physician [19, 20]. In this book, Lanza and Kaski review treatment options available for CSX and propose practical treatment algorithms for the condition (Chap. 27). Successful treatment usually depends on identifying the prevailing pathogenic mechanism and tailoring the intervention to the individual patient. Advice on lifestyle changes and risk factor management–in particular aggressive lipid lowering therapy with statins—should be considered vital components of any therapeutic strategy. A multidisciplinary approach is required in most cases. Briefly, antianginals such as calcium antagonists and β-adrenergic blockers are useful in patients with documented myocardial ischemia or abnormal myocardial perfusion. Sublingual nitrates are effective in approximately 50 % of CSX patients [3]. Little evidence is available in relation to the efficacy of nicorandil, α-adrenergic blockers, trimetazidine, and angiotensin-converting enzyme inhibitors in this setting.

Analgesic intervention with imipramine [21] and with aminophylline [22, 23], has been shown to improve symptoms in patients with chest pain and normal coronary arteriograms. Transcutaneous electrical nerve stimulation and spinal cord stimulation can offer good pain control in some cases. Chapter 32 by Bairey Merz and colleagues is devoted to the management of chest pain and provides useful practical suggestions.

Hormone Therapy

Hormone therapy has been shown to improve chest pain and endothelial function in women with CSX [10]. Estrogen antagonizes the effects of ET-1 and dilates the coronary vasculature. In addition, estrogen modulate pain threshold. Controlled clinical trials have suggested, however, that the risk of developing cardiovascular disease and breast cancer increases in women taking hormone therapy (HT). Thus, although HT has potential cardiovascular benefits, it can also cause harm [24]. The US Preventative Services Task Force has suggested that routine postmenopausal HT should not be advised for the prevention of chronic conditions and women should take an active part in decisions regarding HT. These recommendations apply also to CSX patients. However, HT may be useful in specific cases where a direct relationship exists between estrogen deficiency and CSX symptoms. Several chapters in the book deal with hormones in both pathogenesis and management of CSX. Shufelt and Waldman discuss the management of estrogen deficiency in Chap. 29, whereas Hermsmeyer and Thompson in Chap. 30 develop a new concept regarding the role of progesterone deficiency in CSX. Webb and Collins, in Chap. 28, focus on testosterone.

Psychological Intervention

Psychological intervention may be beneficial for a substantial number of patients, whether or not organic factors are involved [25]. Studies support the role of a structured cognitive behavioral approach to the management of CSX patients with non-ischemic chest pain [25], and this treatment is more likely to be effective if it is begun early after diagnosis.

Physical Training

As a result of physical deconditioning and low pain threshold, CSX patients have an impaired exercise capacity [26]. Physical training improves pain threshold and endothelial function and delays the onset of exertional pain in patients with typical chest pain and normal coronary arteries [26].

Summary

Controversy still exists regarding the pathogenesis and management of CSX. New data have emerged in recent years that provide useful insight regarding pathogenic mechanisms and prognosis of chest pain with normal coronary arteries and the management of these patients. These issues are thoroughly discussed in the book, with the aim of providing a comprehensive picture that can help physicians to identify the prevailing mechanisms and deliver rational and effective management strategies.

Acknowledgments This work was supported by contracts from the National Heart, Lung and Blood Institutes, nos. N01-HV-68161, N01-HV-68162, N01-HV-68163, N01-HV-68164, RO1-HL-073412-01, grants U0164829, U01 HL649141, U01 HL649241, 1 R01 HL092957-01A1, and grants from the Gustavus and Louis Pfeiffer Research Foundation, Danville, NJ, The Women's Guild of Cedars-Sinai Medical Center, Los Angeles, CA, The Ladies Hospital Aid Society of Western Pennsylvania, Pittsburgh, PA, and QMED, Inc., Laurence Harbor, NJ, and the Edythe L. Broad Endowment, Cedars-Sinai Medical Center, Los Angeles, CA, and the Barbra Streisand Women's Cardiovascular Research and Education Program, Cedars-Sinai Medical Center, Los Angeles. JCK's work is supported by St George's University of London, UK.

References

1. Patel MR, Peterson ED, Dai D, Brennan JM, Redberg RF, Anderson HV, Brindis RG, Douglas PS. Low diagnostic yield of elective coronary angiography. N Engl J Med. 2010;362:886–95. Erratum in: N Engl J Med. 2010;363:498.
2. Cannon III RO, Epstein SE. "Microvascular angina" as a cause of chest pain with angiographically normal coronary arteries. Am J Cardiol. 1988;61:1338–43.
3. Kaski JC, Rosano GM, Collins P, et al. Cardiac syndrome X: clinical characteristics and left ventricular function: long-term follow-up study. J Am Coll Cardiol. 1995;25:807–14.
4. Zeiher AM, Krause T, Schachinger V, et al. Impaired endothelium-dependent vasodilation of coronary resistance vessels is associated with exercise-induced myocardial ischemia. Circulation. 1995;91:2345–52.
5. Egashira K, Inou T, Hirooka Y, et al. Evidence of impaired endothelium-dependent coronary vasodilatation in patients with angina pectoris and normal coronary angiograms. N Engl J Med. 1993;328:1659–64.
6. Kaski JC, Cox ID, Crook JR, et al. Differential plasma endothelin levels in subgroups of patients with angina and angiographically normal coronary arteries. Am Heart J. 1998;136:412–17.
7. Cox ID, Botker HE, Bagger JP, et al. Elevated endothelin concentrations are associated with reduced coronary vasomotor responses in patients with chest pain and normal coronary arteriograms. J Am Coll Cardiol. 1999;34:455–60.
8. Kaski JC. Pathophysiology and management of patients with chest pain and normal coronary arteriograms (cardiac syndrome X). Circulation. 2004;109:568–72.
9. Cosin-Sales J, Pizzi C, Brown S, et al. C-Reactive protein, clinical presentation and ischemic activity in patients with chest pain and normal coronary angiograms. J Am Coll Cardiol. 2003;41:1468–74.
10. Kaski JC. Overview of gender aspects of cardiac syndrome X. Cardiovasc Res. 2002;53:620–6.
11. Panting JR, Gatehouse PD, Yang GZ, et al. Abnormal subendocardial perfusion in cardiac syndrome X detected by cardiovascular magnetic resonance imaging. N Engl J Med. 2002;346:1948–53.
12. Buchthal SD, den Hollander JA, Merz CN, et al. Abnormal myocardial phosphorus-31 nuclear magnetic resonance spectroscopy in women with chest pain but normal coronary angiograms. N Engl J Med. 2000;342:829–35.
13. Lanza GA, Giordano A, Pristipino C, et al. Abnormal cardiac adrenergic nerve function in patients with syndrome X detected by [123I] metaiodo-benzylguanidine myocardial scintigraphy. Circulation. 1997;96:821–6.
14. Gulli G, Cemin R, Pancera P, et al. Evidence of parasympathetic impairment in some patients with cardiac syndrome X. Cardiovasc Res. 2001;52:208–16.
15. Rosen SD, Paulesu E, Wise RJ, et al. Central neural contribution to the perception of chest pain in cardiac syndrome X. Heart. 2002;87:513–19.
16. Potts SG, Bass C. Chest pain with normal coronary arteries: psychological aspects. In: Kaski JC, editor. Chest pain with normal coronary arteries: pathogenesis, diagnosis and management. Boston: Kluwer Academic Publishers; 1999. p. 13–32.
17. Jespersen L, Hvelplund A, Abildstrom SZ, Pedersen F, Galatius S, Madsen JK, Jorgensen E, Kelbaek H, Prescott E. Stable angina pectoris with no obstructive coronary artery disease is associated with increased risks of major adverse cardiovascular events. Eur Heart J. 2012;33:734–44.
18. Pepine CJ, Anderson RD, Sharaf BL, Reis SE, Smith KM, Handberg EM, Johnson BD, Sopko G, Bairey Merz CN. Coronary microvascular reactivity to adenosine predicts adverse outcome in women evaluated for suspected ischemia results from the national heart, lung and blood institute wise (women's ischemia syndrome evaluation) study. J Am Coll Cardiol. 2010;55:2825–32.
19. Kaski JC, Valenzuela Garcia LF. Therapeutic options for the management of patients with cardiac syndrome X. Eur Heart J. 2001;22:283–93.
20. Braunwald E, Antman E, Beasley J, et al. ACC/AHA guidelines for the management of patients with unstable angina and non-ST-segment elevation myocardial infarction—executive summary and recommendations. A report of the American College of Cardiology/American Heart Association task force on practice guidelines (Committee on the Management of Patients With Unstable Angina). Circulation. 2000;102:1193–209.
21. Cannon III RO, Quyyumi AA, Mincemoyer R, et al. Imipramine in patients with chest pain despite normal coronary angiograms. N Engl J Med. 1994;330:1411–17.
22. Elliott PM, Krzyzowska-Dickinson K, Calvino R, et al. Effect of oral aminophylline in patients with angina and normal coronary arteriograms (cardiac syndrome X). Heart. 1997;77:523–6.
23. Yoshio H, Shimizu M, Kita Y, et al. Effects of short-term aminophylline administration on cardiac functional reserve in patients with syndrome X. J Am Coll Cardiol. 1995;25:1547–51.
24. Paoletti R, Wenger NK. Review of the international position on women's health and menopause: a comprehensive approach. Circulation. 2003;107:1336–9.
25. Mayou RA, Bryant BM, Sanders D, et al. A controlled trial of cognitive behavioural therapy for non-cardiac chest pain. Psychol Med. 1997;27:1021–31.
26. Eriksson BE, Tyni-Lenne R, Svedenhag J, et al. Physical training in syndrome X: physical training counteracts deconditioning and pain in syndrome X. J Am Coll Cardiol. 2000;36:1619.

Non-Cardiac Chest Pain of Non-Esophageal Origin

2

Cristina Almansa and Sami R. Achem

Abstract

Chest pain is a common clinical problem that can be caused by a broad spectrum of diseases other than coronary artery disease or acid reflux. The diagnosis of non cardiac, non esophageal chest pain can be challenging. The chronic occurrence of chest pain interferes with the daily life routine, mood and productivity of those affected by this condition and therefore implies an enormous socio-economic burden in the community. This chapter offers an overview of some of the most relevant conditions that need to be considered in the differential diagnosis of a patient presenting with chest pain, once that a cardiac and/or an esophageal origin of the symptom has been properly excluded.

Keywords

Chest pain • Epigastric pain • Gastric volvulus • Peptic ulcer • Pneumoperitoneum • Cholecystitis • Choledocolitiasis • Cholangitis • Sphincter of Oddi dysfunction • Pancreatitis • Pancreatic pseudocyst • Pleural fistula • Musculoskeletal pain • Chostochondritis • Tietze syndrome • Precordial catch syndrome • Bornholm disease • Muscle injury • Pseudoangina • Thoracic outlet syndrome • Pneumonia • Pleuritis • Pleural effusions • Pulmonary embolism • Pneumothorax • Pneumomediastinum • Pulmonary arterial hypertension • Anxiety • Panic disorder • Fibromyalgia • Acute aortic syndrome • Sickle cell disease • Drug induced chest pain • Herpes zoster

Introduction

Non-cardiac chest pain (NCCP) can be defined as chest pain resembling angina but without objective evidence of coronary artery disease [1]. NCCP is a source of concern for physicians and patients alike. Chest pain is a common clinical problem. A recent meta-analysis estimated a global prevalence of 13 % (95 % CI 9–16), identifying higher rates in studies performed in Australia, where the pooled prevalence was 16 % (95 % CI 0.2–50) [2]. The prevalence of NCCP has not been studied worldwide, for instance there is lack of

information from certain regions such as Africa or Centro America. The results of different surveys suggest that NCCP affects equally men and women of all ages [2]. A Chinese study reported that the prevalence of NCCP might be inversely related to the socio-economic status but this data has not been confirmed in other populations [3].

Despite the high prevalence of the problem, an Australian study suggests that only a small proportion of patients consult a physician [4]. Interestingly, this survey identified that males were two-times more likely to consult than females, maybe because they were more aware of the risk of heart diseases than their females counterparts [4].

NCCP is also an important cause of work absenteeism and impaired productivity. In Australia 29 % of subjects attending the emergency department for chest pain reported to have missed at least 1 day of work or school in the prior year with and average of 23 days (range 1–240 days) [5].

C. Almansa, MD, PhD (✉) • S.R. Achem, MD, FACP, FACG, AGAF
Division of Gastroenterology, Mayo College
of Medicine, Mayo Clinic Florida,
4500 San Pablo Road, Jacksonville, FL 32224, USA
e-mail: almansa.cristina@mayo.edu; achem.sami@mayo.edu

J.C. Kaski et al. (eds.), *Chest Pain with Normal Coronary Arteries*,
DOI 10.1007/978-1-4471-4838-8_2, © Springer-Verlag London 2013

In addition, up to two thirds of those presenting with NCCP referred some interruption on their daily activities (including work) [6]. Furthermore, NCCP induces a significant impairment of the quality of life comparable to that experienced by patients with cardiac chest pain [6, 7].

The socio-economic burden of NCCP is high, especially as one considers the costs derived from work absenteeism, loss of productivity and the costs of health care. In the USA, it has been reported that almost six million patients visited the emergency department for chest pain in 2007 [8]. In addition patients continue using resources and seeking health care evaluations after being dismissed from hospital. A recent follow up study in a cohort of patients attending the emergency department for chest pain reported that up to 49 % of them visited the emergency department again, 42 % had repeated cardiac evaluations, and 15 % consulted a gastroenterologist. Moreover, the number of health care visits was up to 3 times higher in the subset of patients with chest pain of "unknown origin" than in those with a recognized cause of chest pain [9]. Labeling patients with nonspecific terms such as "non-cardiac, non-esophageal chest pain", "atypical chest pain" or "chest pain of unknown origin" seems to increase their anxiety and frustration leading to continuous medical consultations in search for additional reassurance [6].

The purpose of this chapter is to focus on an overview of some of the non-esophageal causes of chest pain confronting the clinician. Esophageal causes of chest pain and coronary artery disease as source of chest pain are discussed in other sections of this book.

Non-Esophageal Causes of Chest Pain

There is a broad spectrum of diseases, others than coronary artery disease that may cause chest pain, including gastrointestinal, musculoskeletal, pleuro-pulmonary and psychological causes among others (Table 2.1). The diagnostic frequency of each of these entities varies depending on the setting where the epidemiologic study is performed; thus, studies performed in the emergency department show a predominance of cardiac and gastrointestinal diagnoses [9–11], while studies done in primary care settings show predominantly complaints due to musculoskeletal conditions [12, 13].

Gastrointestinal Sources of Chest Pain

Gastric Causes

Epigastric pain is the most frequent form of presentation of gastric disorders. However, pain in the upper abdomen may be difficult to localize and tends to overlap between thoracic

Table 2.1 Causes of NCCP

Gastrointestinal	**Esophagus**
	Gastroesophageal reflux disease
	Motility disorders
	Functional chest pain
	Paraesophageal Hernia
	Eosinophilic esophagitis
	Other causes of esophagitis (infectious, pill, caustic, autoimmune)
	Boerhave syndrome
	Stomach
	Peptic Ulcer
	Gastritis
	Gastric volvulus
	Penetrating/perforated peptic ulcer
	Gall bladder and billiary tree
	Cholecystitis
	Choledocolitiasis
	Cholangitis
	Sphincter of Oddi dysfunction
	Pancreas
	Pancreatitis
	Pancreatic Pseudocyst (extending into the thorax)
	Pancreatic pleural fistula
Musculoskeletal	**Thoracic wall joints**
	Chostocondritis
	Tietze syndrome
	Sternum
	Sternoclavicular syndrome
	Myofascial
	Precordial catch syndrome
	Bornholm disease[a]
	Muscle injury
	Cervical and Thoracic spine
	Pseudoangina
	Thoracic Outlet Syndrome
Respiratory	Pneumonia
	Pleuritis and pleural effusions
	Pulmonary embolism
	Pneumothorax and pneumomediastinum
	Pulmonary arterial hypertension
	Bornholm disease[a]
Psychological	Anxiety and panic disorder
	Others: depression, neuroticism, hypocondria etc.
Malignant disease	Gastrointestinal
	Chest wall
	Pulmonary and pleural
	Breast
	Metastatic disease
Miscellaneous	Fibromyalgia
	Acute Aortic Syndrome
	Sickle cell disease
	Drug induced pain
	Herpes zoster

[a]Bornholm disease may cause musculoskeletal and/or respiratory chest pain

and abdominal organs [14], which explains why sometimes it can be difficult to distinguish from chest pain [15] A recent review suggests that up to 81 % of individuals with endoscopically confirmed peptic ulcer disease present with epigastric pain [16], which has a postprandial pattern that varies depending if the ulcer is located in the stomach (increase of pain after meals) or the duodenum (decrease of pain after meals).

Penetrating or perforating ulcers can also cause epigastric pain that, in case of anterior perforations, rapidly spreads throughout the whole abdomen, accompanied of signs of peritoneal irritation (Fig. 2.1). By contrast, the diagnosis of posterior perforation may be difficult to diagnose or delayed because of the insidious symptoms and lack of physical signs. The symptom most often reported in posterior perforations is abdominal pain that can be epigastric or located in the right upper quadrant, sometimes radiating to the back. The duration and severity increases gradually until it becomes constant and severe [17]. Chest pain and dyspnea have been reported as presenting features of a perforated duodenal ulcer [18]. The radiological demonstration of pneumoperitoneum is a sign of visceral perforation that indicates the need for surgery [17]. Acute and chronic gastritis of infectious, inflammatory or chemical origin can also be cause of epigastric pain [19–23].

Gastric volvulus (Fig. 2.2) occurs when the stomach undergoes axial torsion, often as complication of a paraesophageal hernia but also due to other defects of the esophageal junction or the diaphragm [24, 25]. Acute gastric volvulus is a potential life threatening condition that typically presents with sudden severe chest or abdominal pain, retching without vomiting and dysphagia. In later stages it can cause shock, sepsis and multiorgan failure due to strangulation, ischemia, necrosis and or perforation [26].

Chronic gastric volvulus is more often associated with chronic anemia but may cause recurrent episodes of chest pain that can be erroneously interpreted as coronary disease [27]. The treatment of gastric volvulus is surgical reduction, either open or assisted by laparoscopy [25, 26]. Acute, severe cases who may not be a surgical candidate may be considered for endoscopic decompressive treatment, at least temporarily [28].

Gall Bladder and Biliary Tree

The typical manifestation of symptomatic gallstone disease is biliary pain. Biliary pain is poorly localized in the epigastrium or right upper quadrant and may radiate to the back, right shoulder or the chest. The onset is abrupt, sometimes awakening the patient from sleep. Biliary pain normally occurs as recurrent, not daily, episodes lasting more than 30 min. Though traditionally described as colicky, associated to other unspecific gastrointestinal symptoms and frequently exacerbated after ingestion of fatty meals, recent

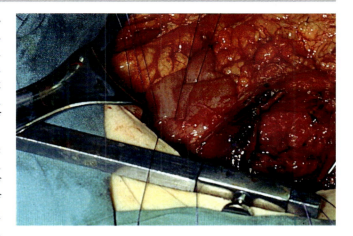

Fig. 2.1 Perforated duodenal ulcer shown at surgery

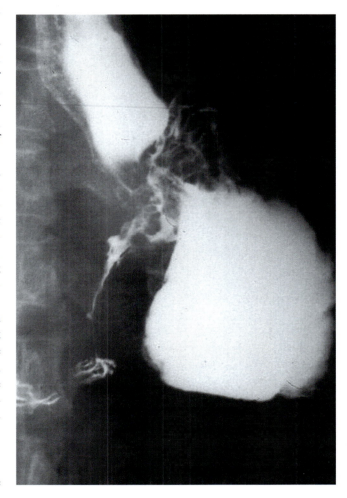

Fig. 2.2 Gastric torsion

definitions characterizes it as steady, accompanied by nausea or vomiting but unrelated to other dyspeptic symptoms, and inconsistently triggered by fatty food intake [29–32]. Pseudoangina pain arising from gallbladder disease has been described worldwide by several authors [33–36].

In patients with NCCP (documented by coronary angiography) the prevalence of gallstone disease by abdominal ultrasound (US) has been reported at 6 % [37]. Reinus and Shady studied the value of gallbladder ultrasound in 52 patients with atypical chest pain referred for biliary ultrasonography. Of those, 12 (32 %) had cholelitasis; and 4 underwent cholecystectomy with complete relief of symptoms [38]. This study underscores the importance of screening for gallstone disease in patients with chest pain.

Biliary pain can be associated with fever in cases of acute cholecystitis, jaundice in cases of choledocholithiasis, and both jaundice and fever (Charcot's triad) in cases of cholangitis [29]. Biliary pain can be also present in absence of gallstones in cases of gallbladder dyskinesia or post-cholecystectomy in patients with Sphincter of Oddi dysfunction [30–32]. The initial diagnostic approach of biliary pain includes abdominal US and pancreatic and liver chemistries; in patients with normal US further steps will depend on the clinical suspicion and may involve the performance of endoscopic ultrasound (EUS), computed tomography (CT), magnetic resonance with cholangiopancreatography (MRCP), cholecistokinin – cholescintigraphy (CCK-CS) and endoscopic retrograde colangiopancreatography (ERCP) with or without Sphincter of Oddi manometry [30, 32].

Pancreatic

Pancreatic pain is often described as epigastric with band-like radiation to the back but can also be localized in the right upper quadrant or involve the entire abdomen. Chest pain may occur in some patients with pancreatitis, especially in cases of thoracic complications [39]. Chest pain from pancreatitis or complications of pancreatitis such as pseudocyst (Fig. 2.3) extending into the mediastinum can also resemble myocardial infarction and even lead to electrocardiographic findings suggestive of ischemia despite a normal coronary angiogram [40–44]. Pneumonia and pleural effusions, most often located in the left hemithorax, are common conditions in acute pancreatitis that most of the times resolve with the improvement of the pancreatic disease. Other potential causes of chest pain in pancreatitis, most often associated to chronic pancreatitis of alcoholic origin, are mediastinal pancreatic pseudocysts and chronic massive pleural effusion secondary to pancreatic pleural fistula [39]. These complications normally arise as consequence of a posterior disruption of the main pancreatic duct into the retroperitoneum and the leakage of pancreatic fluid through the diaphragmatic aortic or esophageal hiatus into the posterior mediastinum [45, 46]. Their initial diagnosis is made by chest radiography and analysis of the pleural fluid, that shows a characteristic increase of amylase (>400 U/L), the diagnosis can be confirmed by an imaging test such as CT, MRCP, or ERCP [46].

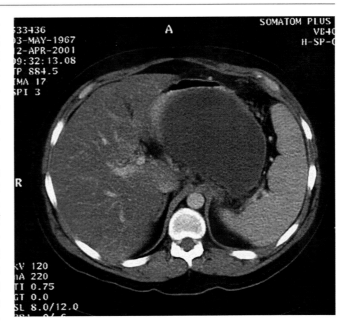

Fig. 2.3 Large pancreatic pseudocyst

Musculoskeletal

Thoracic Wall Joints

Costochondritis

Costochondritis is a common rheumatic condition that represents up to a third of the emergency consultations for acute chest pain [47]. This syndrome can be defined as tenderness of the costochondral and condrosternal joints; and has been termed with different names such as *"costosternal syndrome"*, *"parasternal chondrodynia"* and *"anterior chest wall syndrome"* [48]. The etiology of this syndrome remains unclear, most of the patients report a recent history of repetitive physical activity involving the upper body and/or upper extremity that includes excessive coughing in the course of a respiratory infection [49].

The process often involves multiple sites, normally at the same side of the chest and can affect any of the seven costochondral junctions, though it predominates in the third and fourth ribs. Interestingly, the affected areas do not present external signs of inflammation such as swelling or induration [50], a feature that helps to distinguish it from Tietze's syndrome (discussed later).

The pain has been described as sharp or pressure and increases with the movements of the ipsilateral arm or upper body, and certain situations such as energetic coughing and deep breathing. Chest wall pain is characteristically reproduced by palpation of the affected area; however, this finding though suggestive of atypical chest pain, does not exclude cardiac origin [50]; indeed a study assessing the causes of chest pain in a cohort of 122 patients presenting to the emergency department reported that up to 6 % of those with chostochondritis were also diagnosed with myocardial infarction [47]. The prognosis of chostochondritis is benign and though it can recur, it resolves spontaneously within 1 year [33–36]. The recommended treatment is symptomatic, pain relief with analgesics, anti-inflammatory drugs, rest, physical therapy and reassurance of the benign nature of this process. [50].

Tietze Syndrome

Tietze syndrome is a rare inflammatory disorder that causes non-suppurative swelling of the chostochondral junctions. In contrast with chostochondritis typically affects a single site, most often the second and third ribs, though involvement of the sternoclavicular joint is also possible [49, 50]. Heat and erythema may be present. Tietze syndrome can be secondary to infections, especially in cases of chest wall trauma, rheumatologic disorders and neoplasias [50]. Neoplastic conditions presenting as Tietze syndrome can be primary tumors of the ribs, extensions from a primary process in the vicinity, such as cancers in the pleura, lung or mediastinum or secondary metastatic disease [48, 50–53]. The characteristics of the pain in Tietze syndrome are similar to the described for chostocondritis except for the presence of swelling at the involved site [49]. CT scan can be useful to exclude an infectious or neoplastic process as an underlying cause in suspicious cases [54]. For the most part, the diagnosis is based on history and clinical findings. A recent study suggested that magnetic resonance imaging (MRI) provides a sensitive and reliable tool to confirm the diagnosis [55]. The treatment is similar to that mentioned for chostochondritis.

Ribs

Slipping Rib Syndrome

This syndrome has been referenced in the literature under multiple terms since its first description by Cyriax in 1919 [56]. Synonyms include: "Cyriax syndrome" "rib tip syndrome", "clicking rib", "slipping rib cartilage syndrome", "painful rib syndrome", "nerve nipping", "twelfth rib syndrome", "interchondral subluxation", "displaced ribs" or "traumatic intercostal neuritis" [57, 58]. "Slipping rib syndrome", was first used by Davies-Colley in 1922 [59] and is by far the most popular and quoted term. This syndrome is characterized by tenderness and hypermobility of the anterior ends of the false ribs costal cartilages with the affected rib slipping under the upper rib, displacing and irritating the intercostal nerves [50]. It is estimated that it represents about 5 % of musculoskeletal cases of chest pain in primary care [60] The etiology remains unclear, though some patients refer the origin of the symptoms shortly after or some time after a traumatic event; in other cases there is no inciting

event such as direct or indirect trauma [61]. The pain starts acutely and remains intermittently for minutes with a sharp and stabbing quality; afterwards, the pain is usually described as a dull ache that in some cases can be confused with angina [62]. The diagnosis is clinical and based on the *hooking maneuver* that consists in curving the fingers of the examiner under the affected costal margin pulling gently the rib cage forward and upward, which will reproduce the pain and cause a characteristic "click" [63]. The treatment requires local anesthetic injections or blockage of the intercostal nerve. In some cases, surgical resections of the affected segment may be required [50, 57, 61]. The prognosis is variable with some cases resolving at 3 months with or without treatment and others remaining chronic for years [61].

Sternum

Sternoclavicular Syndrome

This chronic inflammatory disorder of unknown etiology is characterized by pain, swelling and tenderness of the sternoclavicular area. This syndrome has also been termed under different names such as "*sternoclavicular hyperostosis*", "*chronic recurrent multifocal osteomyelitis*" or "*SAPHO*" acronym for synovitis, acne, pustulosis, hyperostosis and osteitis [64–66]. A review of the literature reported that up to 70 % of the patients present with chest pain and 27 % of them also have limited the motion of the shoulder [67]. The diagnosis of this condition is clinical and supported by complementary tests such as bone scintigraphy, which seems to be the best tool to characterize the disease, CT and MRI may also be helpful [65]. There is not a unique treatment of choice, improvement has been reported with a variety of therapies that include, but are not limited to, non steroidal anti-inflammatory agents, corticosteroids, antibiotics, calcitonin, pamidronate, sulfasalazine, colchicine and infliximab [61, 66, 68]. The prognosis of this syndrome seems to be good at long term [68], but a recent series from the UK reported recurrence of the symptoms in up to 41 % of cases [64].

Myofascial

Precordial Catch Syndrome

Also known as *Texidor twinge*, *costalgia fugax* or *devil's grip* was first described by Miller and Texidor in 1955 [69]. The syndrome typically affects young patients, usually under 35 years that complain of intermittent episodes of stabbing non-radiating precordial pain for seconds to a few minutes. [57, 70, 71]. The pain can appear at rest or during mild to moderate exercise. At rest, the pain seems to have a postural origin and disappear after stretching and correcting the position. It also increases with deep breathing and decreases with shallow respiration [49]. The etiology is uncertain but a transient pleural pinching has been suggested as potential cause of the symptoms [70, 71]. It does not require treatment, only explanation and reassurance of its benign nature.

Epidemic Myalgia

This disorder is an acute illness caused by the infection by coxackie B viruses transmitted during outbreaks related to contaminated water [72]. It is also known as *Bornholm disease* or *epidemic pleurodinia*. It may cause pulmonary infiltrates, involve the pleura producing pleural effusions or affect the nearby tissues causing myositis of the abdominal and intercostal muscles and even myopericarditis [73]. It causes intermittent chest pain that increases with deep respiration, frequently associated with fever in young adults [49]. The condition is self limiting and only requires symptomatic treatment.

Muscle Injuries

Soreness and/or tears of the intercostal muscles, pectoralis minor and major can be cause of chest pain in subjects not used to exercise or after intensive muscular activity [57, 74–76]; this is frequent after rowing, heavy lifting or even after a respiratory process associated with intense coughing. Characteristically the pain increases with deep inspiration, upper body movement or coughing and there is tenderness to the palpation of the affected area. Most of the times, the patient recalls the traumatic antecedent, which helps to guide the diagnosis [57]. MRI and US of the affected area can be useful to identify muscular lesions as muscular tears, hematomas or interstitial hemorrhages. Treatment implies rest of the affected muscles, avoiding situations that may exacerbate the pain and use of anti-inflammatory medications for injuries of the intercostal muscles [57], while for lesions of the pectoralis the recommended management includes physical therapy, immobilization of the shoulder and potentially, surgery [76].

Cervical and Thoracic Spine

Pseudoangina

Cervical angina is a cause of chest pain that may resemble cardiac origin, but that arises from severe cervical discopathy with compression of C7 nerve root. The diagnosis is based on the clinical history and confirmed with MRI. Treatment includes physical therapy, muscle relaxants and antiinflammatories [77].

Thoracic Outlet Syndrome

Chest pain can also occur in the thoracic outlet syndrome (TOS), due to compression of the brachial plexus, subclavian artery or vein within the thoracic outlet. There are several entities that may cause TOS, including traumatic and congenital abnormalities such as cervical ribs and other anatomical variations [78].

The main clinical manifestation of this syndrome is pain and paresthesias of the upper extremity ipsilateral to the abnormality. Several cases have been reported where the pain radiates anteriorly to the chest mimicking cardiac angina [79, 80]. An occasional case of a patient with TOS in whom elevation of the arms caused irritation of the brachial plexus leading to coronary spasm by activation of sympathetic nerves has been described [81]. The diagnosis of TOS is complex and requires a high index of suspicion; it will require a detailed history and physical examination including careful palpation and neurovascular examination. The therapeutic management of TOS is controversial, though it has been suggested to attempt conservative measures first, leaving surgery for those with lack of response or patients with neurological symptoms [78].

Fibromyalgia

Fibromyalgia (FM) is a common cause of NCCP. The origin of the pain in these patients may be due to both somatic and visceral hypersensitivity [82]. Studies assessing the prevalence of FM in NCCP, have found variable rates ranging from 2.7 to 25 % [82]. These original studies were based on the classic diagnostic criteria of widespread pain (axial, left and right, and upper and lower segment pain) and tenderness on pressure at 11 of the 18 sites tender points [83]. The new FM criteria proposed by the American College of Rheumatology (ACR) in 2010 [84] and its latest modification in 2011 [85], eliminated the tender points and added the widespread pain index (WPI) and the severity score (SS). The SS evaluates the disturbance produced by other complaints commonly associated to FM such as fatigue, waking unrested and cognitive symptoms, the occurrence of headaches, pain or cramps in the lower abdomen and depression in the last 6 months [85]. The presence of chest pain is evaluated in the WPI that assesses the presence of pain over the last week in any of 19 body sites. The current definition of FM requires a WPI ≥ 7 and a SS ≥ 5 or a WPI 3–6 and a SS ≥ 9. In addition, symptoms must be maintained at the same level of severity for a minimum of 3 months and can not be explained by other disorders [85]. The treatment of FM consists in a multidimensional approach addressing the different symptoms of pain, sleep, mood disorders and concomitant somatic complaints that affect these patients [82].

Pulmonary

Pneumonia

Community acquired pneumonia (CAP) is a common condition that can be fatal in elderly people and patients with important co-morbidity [86]. Classical symptoms of pneumonia may include fever, productive cough, dyspnea and pleuritic chest pain [87]. This later symptom, when present, tends to be localized to the area affected by the pulmonary infection [88]. Atypical symptoms are not infrequent, regardless of the nature of the causal agent, and include arthro-myalgias, headache, and gastrointestinal complaints in up to 30 % of the patients [89]. Pauci-symptomatic presentations are frequent in subjects over 65 years [90]. Diagnostic confirmation of pneumonia requires the identification of pulmonary infiltrate/s at chest radiography; however in some cases, such as in dehydrated patients at early stages of the disease, there maybe few or atypical clinical features [87]. Gram stain and culture of the sputum, when possible, will confirm the microbiological diagnosis and will help guide the antimicrobial treatment. Most patients with CAP can be successfully managed as outpatients; however those at higher risk of complications and mortality must be admitted to the hospital for treatment and close monitoring [91].

Pleuritis and Pleural Effusions

Parietal pleural inflammation is cause of a sharp, unilateral and localized pain that characteristically is aggravated with deep breathing, coughing or any other upper body movements that involve the chest wall. Chest pain can radiate towards the shoulder, neck or the abdomen. Patients with pleuritis, commonly called pleurisy, often present with an exudative pleural effusion, which may be consequence of the increased vascular permeability secondary to the inflammatory process [88]. There are several entities that can lead to parietal pleural inflammation and pleural effusions; the performance of a thoracocentesis to extract and analyze pleural fluid is essential to distinguish between exudates and transudates and guide the differential diagnosis. Characteristically, an exudative pleural fluid contains an increased level of proteins (>0.3 g/dl or ratio pleural fluid protein to serum protein >0.5) and lactate dehydrogenase (LDH) (>200 IU/L or ratio pleural fluid LDH to serum LDH >0.6); a pH <7.2 suggests empyema or pleural malignancies; glucose levels <60 mg/dl is frequent in infections, including tuberculosis but can also denote a rheumathologic origin; amylase levels >200 μg/dl suggest pancreatic disease, rupture of the esophagus or ectopic pregnancy; the presence of blood is indicative of trauma, malignancy or pulmonary embolus; increase levels of tryglicerids (>110 mg/dl) are frequent in tuberculosis or after the rupture of the thoracic duct; overall an increase amount of white blood cells is typical of exudates and specifically the predominance of neutrophils indicates an acute process while the predominance of mononuclear cells suggests chronicity; an increase proportion of lymphocytes is characteristic of tuberculosis or cancer and the rare preponderance of eosinophils is consequence of exposure to asbestos, drugs, parasites or Churg Strauss syndrome [92, 93]. In those cases that remain undiagnosed despite the analysis of the pleural fluid, a pleural biopsy may be indicated. The management of pulmonary effusions will vary depending on the causal entity, though in patients with massive effusions causing dyspnea at rest it will likely include a therapeutic thoracentesis [92].

Pulmonary Embolism

Pulmonary embolism (PE) is consequence of a deep venous thrombosis (DVT) caused by a combination of hypercoagulability, stasis and intimal injury (Virchow's triad) [94]. The most frequent location of DVT is the deep veins of the lower extremities and more rarely in the upper extremities veins (axillary-subclavia veins) [95].

PE classical symptoms are dyspnea of acute onset, chest pain and eventually collapse. Dyspnea is the most common symptom followed by pleuritic chest pain in up to two third of the cases [96]. In the physical exam is relevant the presence of tachypnea and tachycardia, crackles and sometimes an increase in the pulmonary compound of the second sound at cardiac auscultation. A diagnosis of PE is initially suspected in the presence of the classical symptoms and signs in a patient with risk factors for DVT, especially when the arterial oxygen tension (PaO_2) is low. The measurement of circulating D-dimers in plasma can be indicative, but not definitive of PE [97]. An imaging test such as ventilation perfusion scanning, helical CT and pulmonary arteriography will confirm the diagnosis (Fig. 2.4). The treatment of PE requires anticoagulation and if this is not possible, placement of an inferior cava filter.

Pneumothorax and Pneumomediastinum

The diagnosis of pneumothorax implies the presence of air in the pleural space. It may occur spontaneously (primary) or secondary to other underlying conditions such as trauma or pulmonary diseases. Spontaneous pneumothorax usually affects young males that complaint of acute onset of unilateral pleuritic chest pain, cough and dyspnea as a result of spontaneous rupture of apical blebs. Recent reports based on experimental studies suggest that chest pain may be caused by an eosinophilic pleuritis consequence of the air extravasations [88, 98]. The diagnosis is radiographic and involves the demonstration of the visceral pleural line at chest radiography, more evident in expiratory or lateral decubitus radiographic projections (Fig. 2.5) [93].

Pneumomediastinum is characterized by the presence of air in the mediastinum spontaneously or secondary to a trauma. Some causes involve a tear in the esophagus or the rupture of the tracheobronquial tree or alveoli. Clinically, it is characterized by retroesternal chest pain and dyspnea. Severe pneumomediastinum can be accompanied by

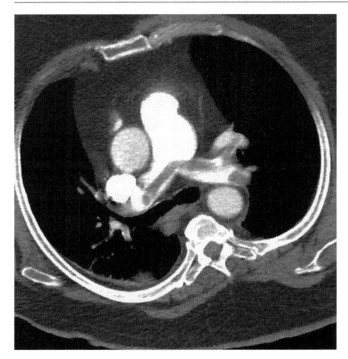

Fig. 2.4 Pulmonary embolism shown using CT

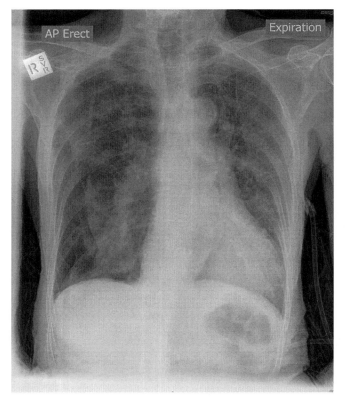

Fig. 2.5 Pneumothorax shown on X-ray

subcutaneous emphysema (air in the subcutaneous tissue), more often located in the chest wall, neck and face. In these cases crepitus can be appreciated on palpation of the affected

areas. The diagnosis of pneumomediastinum is based in the clinical suspicion and confirmed with an imaging test such as CT scan [99]. Both pneumomediastium and pneumothorax may reabsorb spontaneously and therefore may be managed conservatively. In cases of large pneumothorax and tension pneumothorax a chest tube drainage will be required; while those cases of pneumomediastinum secondary to visceral rupture may need surgical repair [93].

Pulmonary Arterial Hypertension

Pulmonary arterial hypertension (PAP) is a rare disorder defined as a mean pulmonary arterial pressure of more than 25 mmHg at rest or 30 mmHg during exercise [100]. PAP can be idiopathic, also known as *primary pulmonary hypertension* or associated with other conditions such as collagen vascular diseases, portal hypertension, congenital cardiac shunts, or HIV infection [101]. The earliest and most common symptom of PAH is the gradual onset of dyspnea after physical exertion. Other symptoms include chest pain, fatigue, syncope, peripheral edema and Raynaud syndrome. The origin of chest pain in these patients is not clear, and it has been attributed to right ventricular ischemia [100] and to pulmonary artery dilation and stretching [88]. Indirect signs of PAP can be seen on a chest radiograph and the electrocardiogram; transesophageal echocardiography, especially if used in combined with Doppler and cardiac catheterization, will confirm the diagnosis and help to establish the prognosis [100]. There is not a curative treatment, but patients can benefit by treatment with diverse therapeutic agents such as anticoagulants, anti-platelet agents, vasodilators, anti-inflammatory drugs and vascular-remodeling therapies [101].

Psychological Disorders

Epidemiological studies suggest that psychological factors play an important role in the pathogenesis of chest pain. Moreover, it seems that patients with NCCP suffer from higher rates of psychological disorders than those with cardiac disease, especially panic disorder (PD). The prevalence of PD in patients with NCCP is about 42 % (range 10–63 %) while the reported rate of PD in patients with CAD is 8 % (range 0–22 %) [102–105].

Other psychological disorders also occur with increased prevalence in patients with NCCP including anxiety, depression, neuroticism, hypochondriac behavior, obsessive-compulsive, avoidant and paranoid disorders [106–110].

Different hypothesis have been proposed to explain the association between psychological factors and chest pain, such an increased tension in the thoracic wall muscles as consequence of anxiety [111], enhanced awareness and monitoring of normal bodily functioning [112], and changes in esophageal motility due to hyperventilation [113, 114].

Longitudinal studies have demonstrated that patients with NCCP and PD present worse psychological outcomes and increased physical impairment that those without PD [115, 116]. A potential association between PD, coronary artery disease and cardiovascular mortality has been suggested [117–119], but this data has not been confirmed in patients with NCCP [116]. Patients with NCCP and PD may have increase rates of suicidal ideation, which could limit their life expectancy [120].

Recognition of potential psychological disorders in patients complaining of chest pain can be essential to improve the outcomes and prognosis of this entity. An algorithm based on gender, age, agoraphobia symptoms and characteristic (quality/location) of pain has demonstrated its usefulness to accurately identify those patients with chest pain presenting a concomitant diagnosis of PD [121].

Malignant Diseases

Chest pain can be precipitated by primary or secondary malignant conditions affecting the pleura and chest wall. Gastrointestinal neoplasias, especially those located in the upper abdomen may also cause epigastric and chest pain.

Chest pain associated with lung cancer is described as isolated, dull and located in the affected side; tumors of the lung apex may cause Pancoast syndrome with pain radiating to the shoulder and chest due to involvement of the braquial plexus; malignant pleural mesothelioma may cause dyspnea and pleuritic pain, that in later stages can be diffuse and of difficult management given the dissemination of the disease through all serous surfaces (pleura and peritoneum) [88].

Chest pain associated with breast cancer is commonly unilateral, persistent and intense; it may radiate to the axilla or arm but otherwise is well localized [122]. Localized mastalgia has been described as an alerting symptom of breast cancer [123], however recent studies suggest that there is not an increased risk of breast cancer in a woman presenting with isolated breast pain [124].

Most common neoplasms of the chest wall are metastatic, especially in the sternum, [74]. Malignant primary chest wall tumors are rare and can arise from any of the structures, bone, cartilage or muscle that constitutes the chest wall. Pain is the most common symptom of both primary and secondary neoplasms of the chest wall. The mechanism of chest pain in chest wall neoplasms is due to periostal or neural invasion. In these cases it is often described as vague, diffuse and confined to a specific area of the thorax. Other frequent symptoms are a palpable mass and in some cases weakness

of the upper extremities caused by compression of the braquial plexus [125].

Miscellaneous

Acute Aortic Syndrome

This term coined by Vilacosta el al. in 2001 [126], comprises an heterogeneous group of disorders that share a common clinical presentation and require urgent care [127]. These entities include: penetrating aortic ulcer, intramural hematoma of the aorta, incomplete aortic dissection and complete aortic dissection. The pathogenesis of each of these disorders is different, though a history of severe hypertension seems to be a common risk factor to all of them. The most frequent and characteristic symptom of this syndrome is the presence of severe chest pain that has been described as pulsating, ripping, tearing or migrating, and whose intensity remains constant from its onset [128]. The radiation of the pain can offer a hint about the topography of the lesion. Injuries of the ascending and thoracic arch, also called proximal or type A, usually radiate to the neck, throat and jaw; while type B, distal or lesions of the descending aorta radiate more often to the back or abdomen. The diagnosis of Acute Aortic Syndrome (AAS) is normally suspected by the symptoms and the combination of normal electrocardiogram findings, signs of aortic dilation in the chest radiograph and an increase in the plasma levels of D-dimers. Diagnostic confirmation usually requires a CT chest, MR, transesophageal echocardiogram and/or aortography. The therapeutic management of the AAS depends mainly on the risk of aortic rupture, and it is normally based on the topography of the lesion. Type A or proximal AAS requires early surgery, while type B patients may be managed conservatively or require surgical or endovascular repair in unstable or complicated cases [129].

Sickle Cell Disease

Sickle cell disease is a hemoglobinopathy due to a glutamic acid to valine substitution at the 6th aminoacid of the β-globin chain of human adult hemoglobin (Hb A). This results in formation of sickle hemoglobin, an autosomal recessive disorder characterized by recurrent vaso-occlusive episodes and hemolytic anemia [130]. Chest pain in these patients can be part of the spectrum of symptoms of the *acute chest syndrome*, one of the most important causes of mortality and hospitalization among patients with sickle cell disease. Chest pain is caused by a combination of fat embolism, infections and vaso-occlusive crisis [131]. However chest pain in the context of sickle cell disease may also be consequence of other cardiopulmonary complications such as pulmonary hypertension and heart disease [130].

Drug-Induced Pain

Cocaine

Chest pain is one of the most common emergency complaints related to the use of smoked, inhaled or injected cocaine. It normally arises within the first hour after cocaine use and remains present an average of 120 min. The pain is more often described as substernal and oppressive and it is frequently associated with shortness of breath and diaforesis [132]. The differential diagnosis of cocaine associated chest pain includes myocardial ischemia, infarction and pulmonary complications such as pneumothorax or pneumomediastinum [133]. Smoked base cocaine, also known as "crack", may cause asthma, interstitial pneumonia or fibrosis and noncardiogenic pulmonary edema. *Crack lung syndrome* is a specific entity associated with the use of smoked base cocaine that often presents with pleuritic chest pain, shortness of breath, cough with carbonaceous sputum and hemoptysis (caused by a combination of pulmonary hemorrhage, pulmonary edema and interstitial disease) [134].

Serotonin Receptor Agonists (Triptans)

The triptans are a group of selective serotonin 5HT 1B/1D receptor agonists that are extensively used for the treatment of moderate-severe migraine. These drugs have all been described to induce chest pain, which is often reported as oppressive and radiated to the throat and/or arms, mimicking myocardial infarction [135, 136]. The pathogenesis of triptans-associated chest pain is not clear. A number of hypothesis have been suggested, including coronary and pulmonary vasoconstriction and changes in esophageal function [137–139]. All triptans may cause chest pain in a dose dependent manner, though this effect seems to be higher with sumatriptan and lower with almotriptan [136, 140].

Other Drugs

Other drugs that may be cause of acute chest pain are aspirin, NSAIDS, ascorbic acid, tetracyclines, ampicilin, clarithromycin, rifampicin, potassium chloride, alendronate and quinidine; The mechanism of production of chest pain in these cases is related to the development pill esophageal injury or pill esophagitis [141].

Herpes Zoster

Thoracic herpes zoster may be a cause of chest pain that occasionally can be misdiagnosed as cardiac angina [10], particularly in those cases when the pain precedes the development of the characteristic skin lesions [142]. Reactivation of varicela zoster has also been recently described as cause of pleuroperdicaditis in an older patient [143]. Despite its rarity this entity needs to be considered in the differential diagnosis of patients with chest pain, especially in those of advanced age or immuno-compromised.

Summary

Chest pain is a common and challenging clinical problem. There is a wide spectrum of clinical conditions that result in chest pain of non-esophageal origin. This chapter offers an overview of some of the common and important causes of non-cardiac, non-esophageal chest pain. A careful clinical history and physical exam frequently provides useful clues to the origin of non-cardiac, non-esophageal chest pain. Recognition of the cause of nonesophageal chest pain may contribute to relieve patients' anxiety and subsequently impact the outcomes.

References

1. Eslick GD. Epidemiology. In: Fass R, Eslick GD, editors. Non cardiac chest pain, a growing medical problem. San Diego: Plural publishing; 2007. p. 1–12.
2. Ford AC, Suares NC, Talley NJ. Meta-analysis: the epidemiology of noncardiac chest pain in the community. Aliment Pharmacol Ther. 2011;34(2):172–80.
3. Wong WM, Lam KF, Cheng C, et al. Population based study of noncardiac chest pain in southern Chinese: prevalence, psychosocial factors and health care utilization. World J Gastroenterol. 2004; 10(5):707–12.
4. Eslick GD, Jones MP, Talley NJ. Non-cardiac chest pain: prevalence, risk factors, impact and consulting -a population-based study. Aliment Pharmacol Ther. 2003;17:1115–24.
5. Eslick GD, Talley NJ. Non-cardiac chest pain: predictors of health care seeking, the types of health care professional consulted, work absenteeism and interruption of daily activities. Aliment Pharmacol Ther. 2004;20(8):909–15.
6. Eifert GH, Hodson SE, Tracey DR. Heart-focused anxiety, illness beliefs, and behavioral impairment: comparing healthy heart-anxious patients with cardiac and surgical inpatients. J Behav Med. 1996; 19(4):385–99.
7. Cheung TK, Hou X, Lam KF, et al. Quality of life and psychological impact in patients with noncardiac chest pain. J Clin Gastroenterol. 2009;43(1):13–8.
8. Niska R, Bhuiya F, Xu J. National Hospital ambulatory medical care survey: 2007 emergency department summary. Natl Health Stat Rep. 2010;26:1–32.
9. Leise MD, Locke 3rd GR, Dierkhising RA, Zinsmeister AR, Reeder GS, Talley NJ. Patients dismissed from the hospital with a diagnosis of noncardiac chest pain: cardiac outcomes and health care utilization. Mayo Clin Proc. 2010;85(4):323–30.
10. Fruergaard P, Launbjerg J, Hesse B, Jørgensen F, Petri A, Eiken P, Aggestrup S, Elsborg L, Mellemgaard K. The diagnoses of patients admitted with acute chest pain but without myocardial infarction. Eur Heart J. 1996;17(7):1028–34.

11. Spalding L, Reay E, Kelly C. Cause and outcome of atypical chest pain in patients admitted to hospital. J R Soc Med. 2003;96(3):122–5.

12. Svavarsdóttir AE, Jónasson MR, Gudmundsson GH, Fjeldsted K. Chest pain in family practice. Diagnosis and long-term outcome in a community setting. Can Fam Physician. 1996;42:1122–8.

13. Buntinx F, Knockaert D, Bruyninckx R, de Blaey N, Aerts M, Knottnerus JA, Delooz H. Chest pain in general practice or in the hospital emergency department: is it the same? Fam Pract. 2001;18(6): 586–9.

14. Munk EM, Drewes AM, Gorst-Rasmussen A, Gregersen H, Funch-Jensen P, Norgard B. Risk of peptic ulcer, oesophagitis, pancreatitis or gallstone in patients with unexplained chest/epigastric pain and normal upper endoscopy: a 10-year Danish cohort study. Aliment Pharmacol Ther. 2007;25(10):1203–10.

15. Barkun A, Leontiadis G. Systematic review of the symptom burden, quality of life impairment and costs associated with peptic ulcer disease. Am J Med. 2010;123(4):358–66.e2.

16. Wong CH, Chow PK, Ong HS, Chan WH, Khin LW, Soo KC. Posterior perforation of peptic ulcers: presentation and outcome of an uncommon surgical emergency. Surgery. 2004;135(3):321–5.

17. Bertleff MJ, Lange JF. Laparoscopic correction of perforated peptic ulcer: first choice? A review of literature. Surg Endosc. 2010; 24(6):1231–9.

18. Assar AN, Sinclair CL, Shrestha DB. Chest pain and dyspnoea resulting from a perforated duodenal ulcer. Br J Hosp Med. 2009; 70(10):599.

19. Madura JA. Primary bile reflux gastritis: diagnosis and surgical treatment. Am J Surg. 2003;186(3):269–73.

20. Yoon WJ, Lee SM, Lee SH, Yoon YB. Gastric anisakiasis. Gastrointest Endosc. 2004;59(3):400.

21. Hokama A, Taira K, Yamamoto Y, Kinjo N, Kinjo F, Takahashi K, Fujita J. Cytomegalovirus gastritis. World J Gastrointest Endosc. 2010;2(11):379–80.

22. Poon TL, Wong KF, Chan MY, Fung KW, Chu SK, Man CW, Yiu MK, Leung SK. Upper gastrointestinal problems in inhalational ketamine abusers. J Dig Dis. 2010;11(2):106–10.

23. Jain R, Chetty R. Collagenous gastritis. Int J Surg Pathol. 2010;18(6): 534–6.

24. Lesquereux-Martínez L, Macías-García F, Ferreirro R, Martínez-Castro J, Gamborino-Caramés E, Beiras-Torrado A. Acute gastric volvulus: a surgical emergency. Rev Esp Enferm Dig. 2011;103(4): 219–20.

25. Chang CC, Tseng CL, Chang YC. A surgical emergency due to an incarcerated paraesophageal hernia. Am J Emerg Med. 2009;27(1): 134.e1–3.

26. Bawahab M, Mitchell P, Church N, Debru E. Management of acute paraesophageal hernia. Surg Endosc. 2009;23(2):255–9.

27. Rathore MA, Andrabi SI, Ahmad J, McMurray AH. Intrathoracic meso-axial chronic gastric volvulus: erroneously investigated as coronary disease. Int J Surg. 2008;6(6):e92–3.

28. Kulkarni K, Nagler J. Emergency endoscopic reduction of a gastric volvulus. Endoscopy. 2007;39 Suppl 1:E173.

29. Wang DQ, Afdhal NH in Feldman: Sleisenger and Fordtran's gastrointestinal and liver disease, 9th ed. Chapter 65. Gallstone disease. Saunders 2010. Online edition, www.mdconsult.com. Accessed on 24 June 2011.

30. Hansel SL, DiBaise JK. Functional gallbladder disorder gallbladder dyskinesia. Gastroenterol Clin N Am. 2010;39(2):369–79.

31. Behar J, Corazziari E, Guelrud M, et al. Functional gallbladder and sphincter of Oddi disorders. Gastroenterology. 2006;130(5): 1489–509.

32. Corazziari ES, Cotton PB. Gallbladder and sphincter of Oddi disorders. Am J Gastroenterol. 2010;105(4):764–9.

33. Kotin VZ, Cheremskoĭ AP, Kutepov SB. Pseudocoronary syndrome in patients with gallbladder pathology. Vestn Khir Im I I Grek. 2007;166(5):96–8.

34. Panfilov BK. Cardialgia in calculous cholecystitis. Klin Med (Mosk). 1974;52(7):60–6.

35. Stojanovic VK, Djaja V, Djordjevic M, Askovic D. Anginal syndrome and cholelithiasis. Lyon Chir. 1969;65(5):735–9.

36. Ravdin IS, Fitz-Hugh T, Wolferth CC, Barbieri EA, Ravdin RG. Relation of gallstone disease to angina pectoris. AMA Arch Surg. 1955;70(3):333–42.

37. Fein AB, Rauch 2nd RF, Bowie JD, Pryor DB, Grufferman S. Value of sonographic screening for gallstones in patients with chest pain and normal coronary arteries. AJR Am J Roentgenol. 1986;146(2): 337–9.

38. Reinus WR, Shady K. Ultrasonographic evaluation of the biliary tree in patients with atypical chest pain. J Clin Ultrasound. 1994;22(1): 17–20.

39. Iacono C, Procacci C, Frigo F, Andreis IA, Cesaro G, Caia S, Bassi C, Pederzoli P, Serio G, Dagradi A. Thoracic complications of pancreatitis. Pancreas. 1989;4(2):228–36.

40. Makaryus AN, Adedeji O, Ali SK. Acute pancreatitis presenting as acute inferior wall ST-segment elevations on electrocardiography. Am J Emerg Med. 2008;26(6):734.e1–4.

41. Albrecht CA, Laws FA. ST. Segment elevation pattern of acute myocardial infarction induced by acute pancreatitis. Cardiol Rev. 2003;11(3):147–51.

42. Jones KS. Non-cardiac chest pain: a variant on Murphy's sign. Non-cardiac chest pain: a variant on Murphy's sign. Med J Aust. 2001;175(7):391.

43. Mettenleiter MW, Lust FJ. Angina pectoris simulated by chronic peripancreatitis and pancreatitis. Am J Dig Dis. 1950;17(1):11–3.

44. Zinther NB, Sommer T. Chest pain caused by pancreatic pseudocyst located in the mediastinum. Ugeskr Laeger. 2007;169(1):61–2.

45. Gupta R, Munoz JC, Garg P, Masri G, Nahman Jr NS, Lambiase LR. Mediastinal pancreatic pseudocyst – a case report and review of the literature. MedGenMed. 2007;9(2):8.

46. Ali T, Srinivasan N, Le V, Chimpiri AR, Tierney WM. Pancreaticopleural fistula. Pancreas. 2009;38(1):e26–31.

47. Disla E, Rhim HR, Reddy A, Karten I, Taranta A. Costochondritis. A prospective analysis in an emergency department setting. Arch Intern Med. 1994;154(21):2466–9.

48. Achem SR, DeVault KR. Noncardiac, nonesophageal causes of chest pain. In: Fass R, Eslick GD, editors. Noncardiac chest pain – a growing medical problem. San Diego: Plural Publishing, Inc; 2007.

49. Fam AG, Smythe HA. Musculoskeletal chest wall pain. Can Med Assoc J. 1985;133(5):379–89.

50. Proulx AM, Zryd TW. Costochondritis: diagnosis and treatment. Am Fam Physician. 2009;80(6):617–20.

51. Pappalardo A, Buccheri C, Sallì L, Nalbone L. Reflexions on the Tietze syndrome. Clinical contribution. Clin Ter. 1995;146(11): 675–82.

52. Uthman I, El-Hajj I, Traboulsi R, Taher A. Hodgkin's lymphoma presenting as Tietze's syndrome. Arthritis Rheum. 2003;49(5):737.

53. Thongngarm T, Lemos LB, Lawhon N, Harisdangkul V. Malignant tumor with chest wall pain mimicking Tietze's syndrome. Clin Rheumatol. 2001;20(4):276–8.

54. Hamburg C, Abdelwahab IF. Reliability of computed tomography in the initial diagnosis and follow-up evaluation of Tietze's syndrome: case report with review of the literature. J Comput Tomogr. 1987;11(1):83–7.

55. Volterrani L, Mazzei MA, Giordano N, Nuti R, Galeazzi M, Fioravanti A. Magnetic resonance imaging in Tietze's syndrome. Clin Exp Rheumatol. 2008;26(5):848–53.

56. Cyriax EF. On various conditions that may stimulate the referred pains of visceral disease, and consideration of these from the point of view of cause and effect. Practitioner (London). 1919;102: 314–22.

57. Gregory PL, Biswas AC, Batt ME. Musculoskeletal problems of the chest wall in athletes. Sports Med. 2002;32(4):235–50.

58. Barki J, Blanc P, Michel J, Pageaux GP, Hachemane-Aourag S, Carabalona JP, Larrey D, Michel H. Painful rib syndrome (or Cyriax syndrome). Study of 100 patients. Presse Med. 1996;25(21):973–6.

59. Davies-Colley R. Slipping rib. Br Med J. 1922;1(3194):432.

60. Verdon F, Herzig L, Burnand B, et al. Chest pain in daily practice: occurrence, causes and management. Swiss Med Wkly. 2008;138:340–7.

61. Wright JT. Slipping-rib syndrome. Lancet. 1980;2(8195 pt 1):632–4.

62. Scott EM, Scott BB. Painful rib syndrome – a review of 76 cases. Gut. 1993;34(7):1006–8.

63. Heinz GJ, Zavala DC. Slipping rib syndrome. JAMA. 1977;237(8): 794–5.

64. Kalke S, Perera SD, Patel ND, Gordon TE, Dasgupta B. The sterno-clavicular syndrome: experience from a district general hospital and results of a national postal survey. Rheumatology (Oxford). 2001;40(2):170–7.

65. Benhamou CL, Chamot AM, Kahn MF. Synovitis-acne-pustulosis hyperostosis-osteomyelitis syndrome (SAPHO). A new syndrome among the spondyloarthropathies? Clin Exp Rheumatol. 1988;6(2):109–12.

66. Hayem G. Valuable lessons from SAPHO syndrome. Joint Bone Spine. 2007;74(2):123–6.

67. Saghafi M, Henderson MJ, Buchanan WW. Sternocostoclavicular hyperostosis. Semin Arthritis Rheum. 1993;22(4):215–23.

68. Hayem G, Bouchaud-Chabot A, Benali K, Roux S, Palazzo E, Silbermann-Hoffman O, Kahn MF, Meyer O. SAPHO syndrome: a long-term follow-up study of 120 cases. Semin Arthritis Rheum. 1999;29(3):159–71.

69. Miller AJ, Texidor TA. Precordial catch, a neglected syndrome of precordial pain. J Am Med Assoc. 1955;159(14):1364–5.

70. Dawson P, Allison DJ. New radiological manifestation of Texidor's twinge. Lancet. 1987;1(8539):978–9.

71. Texidor's twinge. Lancet. 1979;314(8134):133.

72. Ikeda RM, Kondracki SF, Drabkin PD, Birkhead GS, Morse DL. Pleurodynia among football players at a high school. An outbreak associated with coxsackievirus B1. JAMA. 1993;270(18):2205–6.

73. Huang WT, Lee PI, Chang LY, Kao CL, Huang LM, Lu CY, Chen JM, Lee CY. Epidemic pleurodynia caused by coxsackievirus B3 at a medical center in northern Taiwan. J Microbiol Immunol Infect. 2010;43(6):515–18.

74. Habib PA, Huang GS, Mendiola JA, Yu JS. Anterior chest pain: musculoskeletal considerations. Emerg Radiol. 2004;11(1):37–45.

75. Zvijac JE, Zikria B, Botto-van Bemden A. Isolated tears of pectoralis minor muscle in professional football players: a case series. Am J Orthop (Belle Mead). 2009;38(3):145–7.

76. Dodds SD, Wolfe SW. Injuries to the pectoralis major. Sports Med. 2002;32(14):945–52.

77. Wells P. Cervical angina. Am Fam Physician. 1997;55(6):2262–4.

78. Watson LA, Pizzari T, Balster S. Thoracic outlet syndrome part 1: clinical manifestations, differentiation and treatment pathways. Man Ther. 2009;14(6):586–95.

79. Urschel Jr HC, Razzuk MA, Hyland JW, Matson JL, Solis RM, Wood RE, Paulson DL, Galbraith NF. Thoracic outlet syndrome masquerading as coronary artery disease (pseudoangina). Ann Thorac Surg. 1973;16(3):239–48.

80. Godfrey NF, Halter DG, Minna DA, Weiss M, Lorber A. Thoracic outlet syndrome mimicking angina pectoris with elevated creatine phosphokinase values. Chest. 1983;83(3):461–3.

81. Yoshikawa H, Ueno Y, Nakamura N, Tomimoto S. Hands up for angina. Lancet. 1998;352(9129):702.

82. Almansa C, Wang B, Achem SR. Noncardiac chest pain and fibromyalgia. Med Clin North Am. 2010;94:275–89.

83. Wolfe F, Smythe HA, Yunus MB, Bennett RM, Bombardier C, Goldenberg DL, Tugwell P, Campbell SM, Abeles M, Clark P, et al. The American College of Rheumatology 1990 criteria for the classification of fibromyalgia. Report of the Multicenter Criteria Committee. Arthritis Rheum. 1990;33(2):160–72.

84. Wolfe F, Clauw DJ, Fitzcharles MA, Goldenberg DL, Katz RS, Mease P, Russell AS, Russell IJ, Winfield JB, Yunus MB. The American College of Rheumatology preliminary diagnostic criteria for fibromyalgia and measurement of symptom severity. Arthritis Care Res (Hoboken). 2010;62(5):600–10.

85. Wolfe F, Clauw DJ, Fitzcharles MA, Goldenberg DL, Häuser W, Katz RS, Mease P, Russell AS, Russell IJ, Winfield JB. Fibromyalgia criteria and severity scales for clinical and epidemiological studies: a modification of the ACR preliminary diagnostic criteria for fibromyalgia. J Rheumatol. 2011;38(6):1113–22.

86. File TM. Community-acquired pneumonia. Lancet. 2003;362(9400): 1991–2001.

87. Brown PD, Lerner SA. Community-acquired pneumonia. Lancet. 1998;352(9136):1295–302.

88. Brims FJ, Davies HE, Lee YC. Respiratory chest pain: diagnosis and treatment. Med Clin North Am. 2010;94(2):217–32.

89. Marrie JP. Community acquired pneumonia. Clin Infect Dis. 1994;18:501–5.

90. Metlay JP, Schulz R, Li YH, Singer DE, Marrie TJ, Coley CM, Hough LJ, Obrosky DS, Kapoor WN, Fine MJ. Influence of age on symptoms at presentation in patients with community-acquired pneumonia. Arch Intern Med. 1997;157(13):1453–9.

91. British Thoracic Society Standards of Care Committee. British Thoracic Society guidelines for the management of community acquired pneumonia in adults. Thorax. 2001;56 Suppl 4:1–64. iv.

92. Light RW. Pleural effusion. N Engl J Med. 2002;346(25):1971–7.

93. Celli BR. Diseases of the diaphragm, chest wall, pleura and medi-astinum. In: Goldman L, Ausiello D, editors. Cecil text book of medicine, 23rd ed. Chapter 100. Saunders, an imprinted of Elsevier. Philadelphia 2008. Online edition. www.mdconsult.com. Accessed on 11 July 2011.

94. Von Virchow R. Weitere Untersuchungen ueber die Verstopfung der Lungenarterien und ihre Folge. Traube's Beitraege exp path u Physiol (Berlin). 1846;2:21–31.

95. Tapson VF. Acute pulmonary embolism. Cardiol Clin. 2004; 22(3):353–65. v.

96. Stein PD, Terrin ML, Hales CA, et al. Clinical, laboratory, roent-genographic, and electrocardiographic findings in patients with acute pulmonary embolism and no pre-existing cardiac or pulmo-nary disease. Chest. 1991;100:598–603.

97. Ahearn GS, Bounameaux H. The role of the D-dimer in the diag-nosis of venous thromboembolism. Semin Respir Crit Care Med. 2000;21:521–36.

98. Kalomenidis I, Moschos C, Kollintza A, Sigala I, Stathopoulos GT, Papiris SA, Light RW, Roussos C. Pneumothorax-associated pleural eosinophilia is tumour necrosis factor-alpha-dependent and attenuated by steroids. Respirology. 2008;13(1):73–8.

99. Porhomayon J, Doerr R. Pneumothorax and subcutaneous emphy-sema secondary to blunt chest injury. Int J Emerg Med. 2011; 4:10.

100. Gaine SP, Rubin LJ. Primary pulmonary hypertension. Lancet. 1998;352(9129):719–25.

101. Farber HW, Loscalzo J. Pulmonary arterial hypertension. N Engl J Med. 2004;351(16):1655–65.

102. Dammen T, Arnesen H, Ekeberg O, Friis S. Psychological factors, pain attribution and medical morbidity in chest-pain patients with and without coronary artery disease. Gen Hosp Psychiatry. 2004; 26(6):463–9.

103. Huffman JC, Pollack MH. Predicting panic disorder among patients with chest pain: an analysis of the literature. Psychosomatics. 2003;44(3):222–36.

104. Carney RM, Freedland KE, Ludbrook PA, Saunders RD, Jaffe AS. Major depression, panic disorder, and mitral valve prolapse in patients who complain of chest pain. Am J Med. 1990;89(6): 757–60.

105. Carter C, Maddock R, Amsterdam E, McCormick S, Waters C, Billett J. Panic disorder and chest pain in the coronary care unit. Psychosomatics. 1992;33(3):302–9.

106. Bass C, Wade C. Chest pain with normal coronary arteries: a comparative study of psychiatric and social morbidity. Psychol Med. 1984;14(1):51–61.

107. Channer KS, Papouchado M, James MA, Rees JR. Anxiety and depression in patients with chest pain referred for exercise testing. Lancet. 1985;2(8459):820–3.

108. Tew R, Guthrie EA, Creed FH, Cotter L, Kisely S, Tomenson B. A long-term follow-up study of patients with ischaemic heart disease versus patients with nonspecific chest pain. J Psychosom Res. 1995;39(8):977–85.

109. Dammen T, Ekeberg O, Arnesen H, Friis S. Personality profiles in patients referred for chest pain. Investigation with emphasis on panic disorder patients. Psychosomatics. 2000;41(3):269–76.

110. Ho KY, Kang JY, Yeo B, Ng WL. Non-cardiac, non-oesophageal chest pain: the relevance of psychological factors. Gut. 1998;43(1):105–10.

111. Mayou R. Illness behavior and psychiatry. Gen Hosp Psychiatr. 1989;11:307–12.

112. Cheng C, Wong WM, Lai KC, Wong BC, Hu WH, Hui WM, Lam SK. Psychosocial factors in patients with noncardiac chest pain. Psychosom Med. 2003;65(3):443–9.

113. Rasmussen K, Ravnsbaek J, Funch-Jensen P, Bagger JP. Oesophageal spasm in patients with coronary artery spasm. Lancet. 1986;1(8474):174–6.

114. Cooke RA, Anggiansah A, Wang J, Chambers JB, Owen W. Hyperventilation and esophageal dysmotility in patients with noncardiac chest pain. Am J Gastroenterol. 1996;91(3):480–4.

115. Fleet RP, Lavoie KL, Martel JP, Dupuis G, Marchand A, Beitman BD. Two-year follow-up status of emergency department patients with chest pain: was it panic disorder? CJEM. 2003;5(4):247–54.

116. Bull Bringager C, Arnesen H, Friis S, Husebye T, Dammen T. A long-term follow-up study of chest pain patients: effect of panic disorder on mortality, morbidity, and quality of life. Cardiology. 2008;110(1):8–14.

117. Fleet RP, Beitman BD. Cardiovascular death from panic disorder and panic-like anxiety: a critical review of the literature. J Psychosom Res. 1998;44(1):71–80.

118. Gomez-Caminero A, Blumentals WA, Russo LJ, Brown RR, Castilla-Puentes R. Does panic disorder increase the risk of coronary heart disease? A cohort study of a national managed care database. Psychosom Med. 2005;67(5):688–91.

119. Kawachi I, Sparrow D, Vokonas PS, Weiss ST. Symptoms of anxiety and risk of coronary heart disease. The Normative Aging Study. Circulation. 1994;90(5):2225–9.

120. Fleet RP, Dupuis G, Kaczorowski J, Marchand A, Beitman BD. Suicidal ideation in emergency department chest pain patients: panic disorder a risk factor. Am J Emerg Med. 1997;15(4):345–9.

121. Fleet RP, Dupuis G, Marchand A, Burelle D, Beitman BD. Detecting panic disorder in emergency department chest pain patients: a validated model to improve recognition. Ann Behav Med. 1997;19(2):124–31.

122. Preece PE, Baum M, Mansel RE, Webster DJ, Fortt RW, Gravelle IH, Hughes LE. Importance of mastalgia in operable breast cancer. Br Med J (Clin Res Ed). 1982;284(6325):1299–300.

123. Fariselli G, Lepera P, Viganotti G, Martelli G, Bandieramonte G, Di Pietro S. Localized mastalgia as presenting symptom in breast cancer. Eur J Surg Oncol. 1988;14(3):213–15.

124. Smith RL, Pruthi S, Fitzpatrick LA. Evaluation and management of breast pain. Mayo Clin Proc. 2004;79(3):353–72.

125. Shah AA, D'Amico TA. Primary chest wall tumors. J Am Coll Surg. 2010;210(3):360–6.

126. Vilacosta I, Román JA. Acute aortic syndrome. Heart. 2001;85(4):365–8.

127. Lansman SL, Saunders PC, Malekan R, Spielvogel D. Acute aortic syndrome. J Thorac Cardiovasc Surg. 2010;140(6 Suppl):S92–7.

128. Wooley CF, Sparks EH, Boudoulas H. Aortic pain. Prog Cardiovasc Dis. 1998;40(6):563–89.

129. Vilacosta I, Aragoncillo P, Cañadas V, San Román JA, Ferreirós J, Rodríguez E. Acute aortic syndrome: a new look at an old conundrum. Heart. 2009;95(14):1130–9.

130. Rees DC, Williams TN, Gladwin MT. Sickle-cell disease. Lancet. 2010;376(9757):2018–31.

131. Vichinsky EP, Neumayr LD, Earles AN, Williams R, Lennette ET, Dean D, Nickerson B, Orringer E, McKie V, Bellevue R, Daeschner C, Manci EA. Causes and outcomes of the acute chest syndrome in sickle cell disease. National Acute Chest Syndrome Study Group. N Engl J Med. 2000;342(25):1855–65.

132. Hollander JE, Hoffman RS, Gennis P, Fairweather P, DiSano MJ, Schumb DA, Feldman JA, Fish SS, Dyer S, Wax P, et al. Prospective multicenter evaluation of cocaine-associated chest pain. Cocaine Associated Chest Pain (COCHPA) Study Group. Acad Emerg Med. 1994;1(4):330–9.

133. Levis JT, Garmel GM. Cocaine-associated chest pain. Emerg Med Clin North Am. 2005;23(4):1083–103.

134. Haim DY, Lippmann ML, Goldberg SK, Walkenstein MD. The pulmonary complications of crack cocaine. A comprehensive review. Chest. 1995;107(1):233–40.

135. Visser WH, Jaspers NM, de Vriend RH, Ferrari MD. Chest symptoms after sumatriptan: a two-year clinical practice review in 735 consecutive migraine patients. Cephalalgia. 1996;16(8):554–9.

136. Keam SJ, Goa KL, Figgitt DP. Almotriptan: a review of its use in migraine. Drugs. 2002;62(2):387–414.

137. Houghton LA, Foster JM, Whorwell PJ, Morris J, Fowler P. Is chest pain after sumatriptan oesophageal in origin? Lancet. 1994;344(8928):985–6.

138. Foster JM, Houghton LA, Whorwell PJ, Morris J. Altered oesophageal motility following the administration of the 5-HT1 agonist, sumatriptan. Aliment Pharmacol Ther. 1999;13(7):927–36.

139. Maassen VanDenBrink A, Reekers M, Bax WA, Ferrari MD, Saxena PR. Coronary side-effect potential of current and prospective antimigraine drugs. Circulation. 1998;98(1):25–30.

140. Dodick DW. Triptans and chest symptoms: the role of pulmonary vasoconstriction. Cephalalgia. 2004;24(4):298–304.

141. Abid S, Mumtaz K, Jafri W, Hamid S, Abbas Z, Shah HA, Khan AH. Pill-induced esophageal injury: endoscopic features and clinical outcomes. Endoscopy. 2005;37(8):740–4.

142. Ozdemir R, Tuncer C, Güven A, Sezgin AT. A case of herpes zoster misdiagnosed and treated as unstable angina pectoris. J Eur Acad Dermatol Venereol. 2000;14(4):317–19.

143. Ma TS, Collins TC, Habib G, Bredikis A, Carabello BA. Herpes zoster and its cardiovascular complications in the elderly–another look at a dormant virus. Cardiology. 2007;107(1):63–7.

Anisa Shaker and C. Prakash Gyawali

Abstract

Non-cardiac chest pain (NCCP) consists of recurrent angina-type pain unrelated to ischemic heart disease or other cardiac source after a reasonable workup. The most common esophageal cause of NCCP is gastro-esophageal reflux disease (GERD), followed by esophageal motor disorders and esophageal visceral hypersensitivity. Noxious triggers for NCCP include acidic and non-acidic reflux events, mechanical distension and muscle spasm, particularly longitudinal smooth muscle contraction. Functional chest pain of esophageal origin is diagnosed when endoscopy and esophageal physiologic studies (manometry, ambulatory pH/pH-impedance monitoring) do not reveal a source for NCCP. Once a cardiac etiology has been reliably excluded, an empiric proton pump inhibitor (PPI) trial provides a clinically useful and cost effective mechanism for diagnosis of GERD related NCCP. While endoscopy has a limited diagnostic yield because of the high prevalence of nonerosive disease, histopathology may help evaluate for microscopic evidence of reflux and eosinophilic esophagitis. Ambulatory pH or pH/impedance monitoring off PPI therapy assesses for abnormal esophageal acid exposure and reflux association with NCCP events using simple and statistical symptom association probability tests. Esophageal manometry is typically performed concurrent with ambulatory pH monitoring and can identify esophageal dysmotility, some patterns of which may be associated with esophageal hypersensitivity. Acid suppression with a PPI is the first therapeutic measure initiated even prior to investigation in NCCP. Pain modulators (e.g. low dose tricyclic antidepressants) are often the mainstay of therapy in refractory situations. Smooth muscle relaxants (sublingual nitroglycerine, phosphodiesterase-5 inhibitors, and calcium channel blockers) can be used in hypermotility states, although their efficacy has not been conclusively demonstrated in controlled trials. Hypnotherapy, biofeedback, transcutaneous nerve stimulation, and cognitive and behavioral therapy complement pharmacologic therapy, although additional studies are needed; acupuncture may also be of benefit.

Keywords

Non-cardiac chest pain • Gastroesophageal reflux disease • Esophageal motor disorder • Esophageal visceral hypersensitivity • Ambulatory pH monitoring • Esophageal manometry • Proton pump inhibitor • Neuromodulator

A. Shaker, MD • C.P. Gyawali, MD, MRCP (✉)
Division of Gastroenterology, Barnes-Jewish Hospital,
Washington University School of Medicine,
Campus Box 8124 660, South Euclid Avenue,
St. Louis, MO 63110, USA
e-mail: ashaker@wustl.edu; cprakash@wustl.edu

Introduction

Chest pain is a common entity, accounting for a high proportion of office consultations and emergency room visits [1, 2]. The causes of chest pain are multiple and range in severity from merely frustrating to life-threatening. The entity deserving immediate attention and crucial to exclude is cardiac disease, particularly ischemic etiologies, but also non-ischemic disease. Once cardiac etiologies of chest pain have been adequately excluded with cardiology opinion and appropriate diagnostic tests, the focus of further evaluation and management can shift to the entity commonly termed non-cardiac chest pain (NCCP). While routine cardiac testing (stress testing, cardiac catheterization, echocardiography, cardiac MRI) may adequately exclude most active cardiac disease, rare syndromes of intermittent coronary vasospasm or syndrome X may be more difficult to exclude, as is explained in detail elsewhere in the text. Further, cardiac disease can coexist with NCCP, [3]; as many as half of patients with coronary disease may complain of esophageal symptoms [4]. Therefore, patients are recommended to present for urgent evaluation if the character of their symptoms change from those that are designated NCCP after esophageal evaluation.

Non-cardiac chest pain has been defined as recurrent angina-type pain unrelated to ischemic heart disease or other cardiac source after a reasonable workup [5, 6]. A variety of gastroesophageal, other gastrointestinal, pulmonary, musculoskeletal and psychological causes can result in NCCP [7], as described in Chap. 2. The most common origin of NCCP, however, is esophageal. Of the esophageal disorders, gastro-esophageal reflux disease (GERD) dominates the etiology [8, 9]. Less frequent but often cited esophageal causes of chest pain include esophageal dysmotility and esophageal hypersensitivity [10]. This chapter will focus on esophageal pain as a manifestation of NCCP.

Epidemiology

NCCP is a heterogeneous and common disorder with a prevalence ranging from 23.1 % [11] to as high as 33 % in one population based study [1, 12]. The precise epidemiology of esophageal chest pain is difficult to tease out from the bigger category of NCCP, but reports in the literature are likely representative of esophageal pain since this constitutes the bulk of NCCP. Gender prevalence of NCCP is similar although some studies suggest that women tend to seek out medical care for symptoms more frequently than men [1]. Atypical GERD symptoms such as chest pain may also become more prevalent during pregnancy [13]. There is an inverse relationship between the prevalence of NCCP and age [6, 12]. This is likely related to the fact that the esophagus is less sensitive to noxious stimuli with increasing age, and triggers such as reflux events may not invoke as much sensitivity or hypersensitivity as in younger individuals [14–16]. There is a strong link between esophageal pain and affective disorders. Hence, patients with NCCP are also likely to manifest psychological comorbidities such as panic disorder, depression, somatization, and anxiety [6, 17].

Although studies evaluating the cost of NCCP are limited, the economic impact of NCCP cannot be underestimated. Chest pain in general is a cause of multiple outpatient visits, accounting for 2–5 % of emergency room visits, frequent hospitalizations, and often dissatisfaction with provided care [6]. Occupational impairment and work absenteeism rates as high as 29 % have been reported [6, 18]. It is thought that as many as 200,000 new cases of NCCP are diagnosed each year in the US. Most of these patients continue to worry about a sinister cardiac etiology for their pain, sometimes despite documentation of a clear relationship between esophageal events and chest pain. The psychological associations, particularly anxiety and panic disorder, can serve to propagate anxiety and stress, both of which increase physical and psychological comorbidity and health care utilization.

Categories of Esophageal Chest Pain

GERD Related Chest Pain

Gastro-esophageal reflux disease (GERD) is the most common cause of NCCP, accounting for up to 60 % of patients with NCCP [6, 19]. GERD-related NCCP resembles the pain of angina, with squeezing/burning in the substernal location and radiation to the neck, arms or back. This discomfort may persist only a few minutes or last for hours, and may continue intermittently for days [7]. The pain may be worse post-prandially, in the supine position, after exercise, or during emotional stress. Strenuous exercise may initially provoke typical GERD symptoms such as heartburn and regurgitation, which may then in turn lead to NCCP. The presence of esophageal symptoms such as heartburn, dysphagia, and regurgitation can help distinguish NCCP from cardiac angina [17]. There is significant overlap of symptoms, however, and distinguishing the two based on clinical history alone is challenging and not recommended. Patients' description of heartburn and chest pain can overlap, and degree of pain perception can influence symptom intensity and interference with day to day activities. In the setting of GERD, predisposition to abnormal central processing of afferent data may lead to triggering and propagation of chest pain as a symptom, and this can be modified by cognitive and psychological comorbities (Fig. 3.1).

In patients naïve to antisecretory therapy, the likelihood of documenting esophageal erosive changes on upper endoscopy is significantly lower in NCCP (15–20 %) compared to typical reflux presentations (50–60 %) [17]. The incidence of esophagitis goes down even further in patients treated with proton pump inhibitors (PPIs), making endoscopy an unreliable study in diagnosing GERD in NCCP [2, 6, 17]. Endoscopy may have value if visual and histopathologic evidence of Barrett's esophagus is found, indicating a high likelihood of

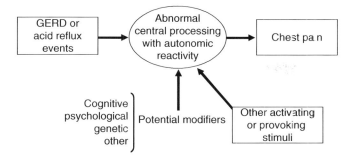

Fig. 3.1 Putative mechanisms by which gastroesophageal reflux disease can trigger chest pain. In patients predisposed to abnormal central processing of peripheral stimuli, reflux events can trigger the perception of chest pain. There may be associated autonomic reactivity, manifesting as dysmotility, inherent to abnormal central processing, and therefore a potential marker of this visceral hypersensitivity pattern. Comorbid cognitive and psychological factors are known modifiers of this process, and genetic predispositions are being identified, but other yet unknown modifiers could exist. In addition to reflux events, other esophageal physiologic or pathologic events could participate in activating or potentiating the process

concurrent GERD and a need for PPI therapy. Histopathology has value in determining nonerosive reflux disease, and in excluding eosinophilic esophagitis, which can also present with chest pain or heartburn. Newer endoscopic modalities such as narrow band imaging may help identify mucosal and vascular changes associated with reflux disease [20, 21]. Although endoscopy is typically the first test performed, the low yield typically leads to further esophageal testing, particularly ambulatory pH or pH/impedance monitoring. When performed off antisecretory therapy, both quantitation of esophageal acid exposure and assessment of correlation between chest pain and reflux events have value in determining the etiology of NCCP. Prolonging the pH recording period beyond the traditional 24 h study using wireless pH monitoring may further improve the diagnostic yield. Prolonged pH monitoring takes into account day-to-day variation in acid exposure while evaluating GERD evidence, and allows more symptoms to develop for symptom reflux correlation [22–24]. The likelihood of documenting abnormal parameters on ambulatory pH studies ranges from 25 to 60 % [7].

Esophageal Dysmotility Related Chest Pain

Up to 30 % of patients with NCCP are reported to have esophageal motor abnormalities including diffuse esophageal spasm, "nutcracker" esophagus, and hypertensive LES [18]. Early balloon distension studies have documented higher sensitivity to lower volumes of balloon distension in NCCP patients compared to healthy normal volunteers in this setting [25]. Graded balloon distension studies have shown lower sensory threshold, and higher degrees of pain to similar balloon distension pressures compared to controls [26]. A positive correlation

exists between amplitude of esophageal body contraction and intensity of pain perception, suggesting that hypercontraction is associated with hypersensitivity [27]. Using impedance planimetry, which assesses cross sectional area in the esophagus, muscle reactivity was noted at a lower threshold on balloon distension in NCCP patients compared to controls [26]. This hypersensitivity seen in spastic disorders may further translate into incomplete symptom relief with typical antireflux treatments (including surgery) when these disorders overlap with GERD [28]. Therefore, although a definitive causal relationship between manometric abnormalities and chest pain has not been conclusively established, hypercontraction appears to be associated with hypersensitivity in the esophagus.

Spontaneous and edrophonium induced sustained longitudinal muscle esophageal contractions, evaluated by ultrasonography have been demonstrated to be associated with chest pain [3, 29]. Although sustained esophageal contractions are associated with pain, most patients with NCCP have normal esophageal motility [6]. In those patients with manometric abnormalities, there is no consistent relationship between dysmotility and reports of chest pain. Despite this, the esophagus has been described to be stiff and noncompliant in NCCP patients, especially in the setting of hypercontractile states such as 'nutcracker esophagus' [26, 30]. Blocking reactivity and relaxing the wall with atropine, however, does not remove the hyperalgesia, suggesting that the relationship between hypercontraction and hyperalgesia is more complex [31]. Chest pain is also reported with extreme motor disorders such as achalasia and diffuse esophageal spasm, but these account for only a small proportion of subjects with NCCP [6]. Hypercontractile and spastic disorders represent disorders of esophageal inhibitory nerve function [32, 33] and the possibility remains that hypersensitivity leading to NCCP is an epiphenomenon seen with esophageal inhibitory nerve dysfunction [18]. Psychiatric comorbidities may also participate in symptom perception and reporting in this cohort of patients, as the prevalence of generalized anxiety disorder and major depression are higher in patients with nonspecific spastic disorders of the esophagus (40–42 %) than in NCCP patients in general (14–24 %) [34]. There is enough evidence in the literature to recommend esophageal motility testing in patients with unexplained NCCP, as the finding of a spastic process will prompt consideration of esophageal hypersensitivity as a mechanism for symptoms.

Esophageal Hypersensitivity

Esophageal hypersensitivity overlaps with the above two categories described, and may also overlap with functional chest pain. Esophageal hypersensitivity can be defined as symptoms arising from unexpected reaction to physiological stimuli, and/or exaggerated response to pathological stimuli.

Psychiatric comorbidity may contribute to the exaggerated symptom perception in these patients. There is data to suggest that stressful situations, either simulated or in real life, are associated with heightened esophageal symptom perception [35, 36]. However, benefit in terms of relief of NCCP may not be evident despite change in anxiety or depression ratings, correction of abnormal motility pattern or correction of visceral hypersensitivity. Somatization state and trait also form a subset of subjects with esophageal hypersensitivity and functional chest pain, and can frequently be identified on the basis of symptom check lists and multiple functional diagnoses [37].

Eosinophilic Esophagitis

Eosinophilic esophagitis (EoE) is a distinct clinico-pathologic disorder characterized by PPI refractory esophageal symptoms in combination with dense esophageal eosinophilia. Population based studies suggest an increase in the incidence of EoE over the past 30 years with a prevalence of 55 per 100,000 persons [38]. Affected children and adults are more likely to be male [39, 40]. The clinical presentation of EoE varies with age. In adults, solid food dysphagia and food impaction are the most commonly observed symptoms [41] while in children the range of manifestations are more broad and include feeding difficulties, abdmoninal pain, dysphagia, and vomiting. As recognition of EoE as a disorder has increased, there has a been a corresponding increase in reports of NCCP in association with EoE [41, 42]. A recent retrospective study supports the role for endoscopy with esophageal biopsies especially in males with recurrent unexplained chest pain [42].

Infectious Esophagitis

Infectious esophagitis can result from bacterial, viral, fungal, or parasitic organisms. Although immunocompetent individuals without predisposing factors can develop these infections, infectious esophagitis typically occurs in immunocompromised states, including chemotherapy, transplantation, and HIV infection. Diabetes and recent antibiotic are also predisposing factors. The most commonly described organisms are candida, herpes simplex virus (HSV), and cytomegalovirus (CMV). Less commonly reported agents include cryptosporidium and mycobacterium avium complex (MAC). Although endoscopic and histologic appearances are specific to the infectious agent, clinical manifestations are similar and include dysphagia and/or odynophagia. Odynophagia can be particularly prominent with HSV esophagitis, and may be interpreted as NCCP. It is important to note that HSV esophagitis can also occur in an immunocompetent and

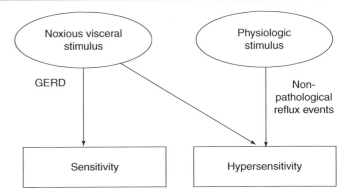

Fig. 3.2 Concepts regarding esophageal sensitivity and hypersensitivity. Noxious peripheral stimuli trigger sensitivity, an expected and physiologic phenomenon. In susceptible individuals, the same noxious stimuli, or in some instances, normal physiologic stimuli can generate an exaggerated perceptive reaction. This exaggerated response is termed hypersensitivity

otherwise healthy host. Candida esophagitis can also present with retrosternal chest pain [43]. In general, infectious esophagitis has a shorter temporal profile compared to other NCCP etiologies, and may be self limited.

Functional Chest Pain

Many patients with NCCP have esophageal visceral hypersensitivity concurrent with esophageal dysmotility or GERD [6]. However, there are patients with esophageal chest pain that have normal endoscopy, normal esophageal motility testing and normal ambulatory pH/impedance testing. This pattern is recognized as functional chest pain of presumed esophageal origin (Rome II), defined as "at least 12 weeks, which need not be consecutive, in the preceding 12 months of midline chest pain or discomfort that is not of burning quality; and absence of pathologic gastro-esophageal reflux, achalasia, or other motility disorder with a recognized pathologic basis" [44]. Visceral hypersensitivity, which has been defined as enhanced conscious perception of a visceral stimulus regardless of the stimulus intensity, is thought to play a pathogenic role in functional NCCP [44] (Fig. 3.2). In addition, up to 75 % of patients with NCCP reportedly have some psychological co-morbidity, most commonly panic disorder, anxiety, somatization, or depression [17]. While affective disorders, stress, and luminal events such as mucosal inflammation may act as triggers, these are often not evident, and may not be required for the initiation or propagation of functional chest pain. Core abnormalities are thought to include distorted central processing of peripheral stimuli; autonomic reactivity and dysregulation may contribute, and may be responsible for the epiphenomena seen in the form of motor dysfunction in some patients [45] (Fig. 3.3).

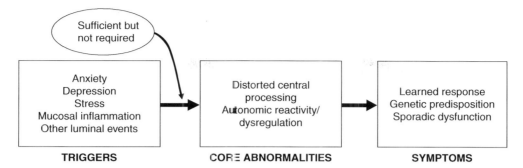

Fig. 3.3 Factors contributing to hypersensitive and functional mechanisms of chest pain. The core abnormalities focus on abnormal central processing of peripheral inputs, which in turn are provoked or triggered by physical luminal events and/or cognitive and psychological events. Once symptoms develop, they may be propagated by the learned response that develops, and therefore can persist long after the triggers resolve. While many cases seem to be sporadic events, genetic predispositions probably exist, and are currently being investigated

Pathophysiology

The mechanisms underlying esophageal chest pain have not yet been definitively elucidated. Animal and human studies have demonstrated that several types of esophageal stimuli can result in chest pain, including acid exposure, mechanical distension, and muscle spasm. How the esophagus responds to these stimuli is an ongoing area of research.

The similarity of esophageal pain to cardiac pain is not altogether surprising given the anatomic proximity of the esophagus and heart and their shared innervation. There is convergence of cardiac and esophageal sensory afferent fibers on the same neurons of the spinal dorsal horn in the cervical and thoracic spinal cord [46, 47]. Areas of pain perception, both primary perception and radiation, are remarkably similar for esophageal and cardiac pain [48]. For instance, radiation to the left shoulder can be seen in 23 % and to the left arm in 18 % of esophageal chest pain [48]. Some characteristics of pain, however, are suggestive of esophageal origin, such as prolonged duration of pain, prompt relief with antacids, pain waking patients' up from sleep, and associated esophageal symptoms such as dysphagia, odynophagia, heartburn and regurgitation. Both esophageal and cardiac pain may be associated with similar high scores when tested for psychosocial factors (stress, anxiety, depression), clinical pain responses, and pain coping strategies, leading some to believe that the abnormal psychological measures may be inherent to the presence of pain rather than caused by pain [49].

The association of chest pain with acid reflux events has been demonstrated in multiple studies [6]. The relationship between NCCP and GERD is further supported by symptom resolution with anti-secretory therapy [6]. The association of GERD with chest pain is likely multi-factorial, however, and several mechanisms underlying this relationship have been proposed. GERD induced NCCP may be a consequence of activation of esophageal wall nociceptors (chemo- and mechano-receptors) in response to chemical and thermal stimulation, and esophageal wall stretch [7]. These signals are transmitted peripherally and centrally. Acid reflux may also manifest as chest pain in these patients by provoking a hypersensitivity response via peripheral sensitization, whereby there is a decrease in the response threshold and a heightened perception to esophageal chemo- and mechano- stimulation [7]. Alternatively, there may be central sensitization at the level of neurons in the spinal cord and brain [1] (Fig. 3.2).

Esophageal acid has also been shown to excite esophageal vagal and spinal sensory afferent fibers via activation of proton-gated ion channels [50]. Candidate receptors for acid sensitivity in the esophagus include the vanilloid receptor 1 (TRPV1) and acid sensing ion channels (ASIC). TRPV1 is expressed by esophageal sensory neurons and is activated by noxious heat, acid pH and ethanol. Upregulation of this acid sensing receptor in esophageal sensory nerve fibers has been proposed as a potential mechanism of esophageal hypersensitivity in NCCP [51]. A reduction in acid related coronary artery flow or a neural cardio-esophageal reflex, has also been proposed as mechanism of acid related NCCP [3, 6, 7, 52]. Acid perfusion has been shown to reduce coronary artery flow in patients with syndrome X; an effect not seen in the denervated heart of heart transplant recipients. Syndrome X, also known as microvascular angina, is characterized by a typical angina symptoms, a positive stress test, and normal coronary angiogram [1].

Although motility abnormalities have been described in patients with non-GERD related chest pain, the significance of these findings in the pathogenesis of chest pain remains unresolved [1]. Esophageal muscle thickness in the absence of esophageal motility abnormalities has been implicated in the pathogenesis of NCCP [6]. There also appears to be a correlation between spontaneous and induced sustained esophageal longitudinal muscle contractions and NCCP [3, 29].

Heightened perception of esophageal acid events, provocation with cholinergic agonists and balloon stimulation under experimental conditions have all been demonstrated in patients with NCCP [18]. Therefore, peripheral sensitization has been proposed as a mechanism contributing to chest pain in patients with esophageal hypersensitivity. Acid reflux may sensitize esophageal afferent pathways to stimuli, lowering the threshold at which patients perceive otherwise normal esophageal distention [1]. Peripheral sensitization is thought to be the primary contributor of pain hypersensitivity at the injury site, or primary hyperalgesia [53]. Central sensitization with an increase in the excitability of spinal cord neurons and enhanced cerebral processing of esophageal sensory input have also been proposed as mechanisms contributing to chest pain in patients with esophageal hypersensitivity [1, 54]. Secondary hyperalgesia or pain sensitivity that affects not only the site of injury but also the surrounding healthy tissue is thought to result from central sensitization [53].

A unified pathophysiologic model of symptom triggering is depicted in Fig. 3.3. The core abnormality is likely a disturbance in central processing of peripheral stimuli; abnormal autonomic regulation related to this potentially causes the epiphenomenon of hypermotility noted on esophageal manometry in some situations. In addition to physical triggers (chemo- or mechano-receptor stimulation), cognitive and psychological comorbidities may contribute to symptom generation and propagation. A learned response may result in persistent symptoms despite improvement or resolution of the physical or psychological trigger. Candidate gene studies, genome wide association studies and whole genome sequencing are being actively researched in an attempt to identify genetic polymorphisms that would identify a predisposing phenotype [55].

Diagnosis

Given that patient history is not sufficient to distinguish between cardiac and non-cardiac sources of chest pain, initial diagnostic tests should be focused on evaluation of cardiac disease (stress test, angiogram). Once a cardiac etiology has been reliably excluded, esophageal causes of chest pain can then be evaluated (Table 3.1).

Proton Pump Inhibitor Test

The PPI test, a short course of twice a day proton-pump inhibitor, is a sensitive, specific, and cost-effective method of simultaneously diagnosing and treating GERD related NCCP [7]. A meta-analysis showed that the sensitivity and specificity of the PPI test were 80 and 74 % respectively [56]. The original PPI test consisted of omeprazole administered orally in the dose of 40 mg in the morning and 20 mg in the evening before meals for a 7 day period. Since chest pain episodes are less frequent compared to heartburn, there have been suggestions that a PPI trial for NCCP needs to last longer, perhaps a month.

Table 3.1 Typical investigative procedures performed on patients with suspected esophageal chest pain

Clinical	PPI test
	Upper endoscopy with biopsy
	Esophageal manometry (preferably high resolution manometry)
	Ambulatory pH or pH impedance monitoring (off PPI)
	Barium studies (less of a role)
	Psychological assessment when appropriate
Research	Balloon distension studies
	Acid perfusion studies (Bernstein test)
	Impedance planimetry
	High frequency ultrasound
	Multimodal stimulation
	Esophageal evoked potentials
	Functional MRI

PPI proton pump inhibitor, *MRI* magnetic resonance imaging

Response seems to mirror that seen with the original studies on non-selected GERD, ranging from 71 to 95 % in randomized controlled studies [8, 19]. However, response or lack thereof may not be conclusive for establishing or refuting GERD. In one prospective randomized control trial, as many as 39 % of NCCP patients without GERD parameters on ambulatory 24 h pH study had a response to PPI therapy [8]. Further, meta-analysis of a short-term PPI treatment in non-selected GERD demonstrated a specificity of only 54 % for a diagnosis of GERD. This study, however, was hampered by limited information on PPI dose and duration. The observed clinical benefit in patients without objective GERD parameters may represent alternate conditions potentially triggered by reflux events including esophageal hypersensitivity, eosinophilic esophagitis or placebo effect [57].

There is data to suggest that in subjects presenting with chest pain and normal coronary angiography, an approach that starts with empirical antisecretory treatment provides significant cost saving, both in the early follow up period, and after 1 year of follow up, compared to approaches that start with extensive gastrointestinal investigation [58]. Despite the cost savings, the proportion of patients with symptom relief was similar on follow up [59]. Given the ready availability of PPI therapy, including generic formulation, its non-invasive nature, and ultimately a cost-saving approach, a short course of PPI therapy to determine response is reasonable before proceeding with more invasive diagnostic evaluation. Endoscopy for histopathology to evaluate for eosinophilic esophagitis and perhaps Barrett's esophagus is reasonable at this stage, regardless of the outcome of the PPI trial. In most secondary and tertiary referrals, a PPI trial and endoscopy would have been performed before referral. In patients unresponsive to PPI therapy, further diagnostic tests can be considered.

Ambulatory pH Monitoring

Interpretation of esophageal pH monitoring in NCCP continues to evolve. Of the available diagnostic tests, pH monitoring is probably the most helpful in demonstrating a relationship between acid exposure and symptoms in patients with NCCP. Ambulatory pH monitoring can be performed using the traditional catheter based system, or the newer wireless system. Traditional pH catheters typically have two recording sites 15 cm apart, and are placed transnasally with the distal recording site positioned 5 cm proximal to the top of the lower esophageal sphincter (LES) as determined by esophageal manometry. Newer catheters combine pH and impedance, such that impedance electrodes are positioned both proximal and distal to the pH recording sites. The advantage of impedance monitoring is that refluxates can be detected irrespective of pH. With wireless pH monitoring, a pH recording capsule is attached to the esophageal wall 6 cm proximal to the endoscopically identified squamocolumnar junction using a transoral delivery device, to correspond to the typical positioning of the pH catheters 5 cm above the LES. Using a correction factor, the transoral wireless delivery system can be used with manometrically measured LES distance from the nostril.

Typically, objective measurement of pathologic reflux is determined by acid exposure time or AET, defined as the percentage of time esophageal pH is <4 during a 24 h period. To determine abnormal AET, especially in the setting of an incomplete response to PPI therapy, ambulatory pH testing needs to be performed off anti-reflux therapy [9]. Threshold values for AET range from 4.0 to 5.3 %; higher thresholds are recommended for wireless pH monitoring.

Analysis of pH monitoring includes assessment of symptom reflux association to determine if symptoms can be explained by reflux disease. Many reflux events fail to generate symptoms, and all symptoms may not correlate with reflux events. Traditionally, to designate association with a reflux event, the symptom needs to occur within 2 min of the reflux event. Tests and indices have been developed to confer objectivity to symptom reflux association. The simplest of these tests is the symptom index (SI), which describes the proportion of reported symptom events that correlate with esophageal acidification (pH<4.0), expressed as a percentage. A value $\geq$50 % indicates positive symptom correlation. The SI can be unreliable with low diagnostic yield when symptoms are infrequent [60], but may have value in designating confidence in symptom reflux associations, particularly when other GERD parameters (such as AET and symptom association probability) are also abnormal. Symptom sensitivity index (SSI) is a rarely used test, depicting the ratio of symptoms associated with reflux episodes to the total number of reflux episodes. Symptom associated probability (SAP) is used more often to assess the likelihood

of chance association between symptom and reflux events, using a statistical approach. The entire duration of the pH study is divided into 2 min segments. Each segment is assessed for the presence or absence of reflux events and symptoms. A two by two table is generated with the data, representing sums of four possible combinations, symptom plus reflux, symptom and no reflux, no symptom and reflux, and no symptoms and no reflux. A Fisher's exact test is applied to generate a p value, which suggests less likelihood of chance association if <0.05 [22]. An alternate statistical test, the Ghillebert Probability Estimate (GPE), calculates a similar p value by summing up partial probabilities from data routinely collected during an ambulatory pH study, without need for determining 2 min intervals [22]. In combination with an abnormal AET, a positive symptom association probability has the best value in designating a GERD etiology in NCCP [6, 9]. The SAP has been shown to be independently predictive of symptomatic response to anti-reflux therapy (medical therapy and anti-reflux surgery) in NCCP [9]. Similar symptom association parameters can be applied to pH-impedance monitoring.

If ambulatory pH testing results are normal, other causes of NCCP (esophageal dysmotility, hypersensitivity, psychological co-morbidities) are typically pursued [6, 7].

Endoscopy

Upper endoscopy has limited sensitivity in the evaluation of NCCP, since the majority of individuals with GERD related NCCP have non-erosive disease [60]. Most patients with NCCP undergo endoscopy at some point in their work up. The likelihood of finding erosive esophagitis ranges from 15 to 25 % in symptomatic NCCP patients prior to PPI therapy [8, 17] which decreases further after PPI therapy. However, there may be some value in performing an upper endoscopy. When endoscopic evidence (visual and histopathologic) of Barrett's esophagus is found, the likelihood of GERD is high and PPI therapy is warranted, although this may not fully explain chest pain in all instances. Endoscopy is useful in diagnosing or excluding infectious esophagitis. This may be particularly relevant in acute onset of severe chest pain, which can be seen with herpes esophagitis. Odynophagia and dysphagia can coexist in this setting. Infectious esophagitis is frequently identified in immunocompromised patients, but herpes esophagitis can occur in immunocompetent patients as well [43]. Endoscopy also allows for evaluation and exclusion of eosinophilic esophagitis as a cause for esophageal symptoms. Typical endoscopic findings include linear furrows, circumferential ridging and narrowing, and exudates, although the esophagus can visually appear normal. Biopsies are recommended from both proximal and distal esophagus. Finally, upper endoscopy is also indicated when alarm symptoms (dysphagia, anemia, bleeding, weight loss) are present; lack of response to PPI therapy can be considered an alarm symptom prompting endoscopy.

Manometry

Esophageal manometry is typically considered when structural and mucosal etiologies for NCCP have been excluded, since esophageal motor disorders may be associated with esophageal hypersensitivity. From a practical standpoint, manometry is performed concurrent with ambulatory pH monitoring, especially when catheter based pH or pH-impedance tests are performed, since placement of the pH catheter requires manometric measurement of the distance to the LES.

Prominent motor disorders such as achalasia and esophageal hypermotility (esophageal spasm, nutcracker esophagus) may have an important chest pain component. However, these disorders represent a small proportion of patients with NCCP [60]. With the advent of high resolution manometry (HRM), manometric characteristics have been identified that may have value in the evaluation of NCCP. For instance, exaggerated smooth muscle contraction may be identified by merging together of smooth muscle contraction segments, and increased vigor of contraction as measured by the distal contractile integral (DCI); this can be associated with chest pain predominant presentations [61]. A lesser version of this, a shift in contraction vigor to the distal smooth muscle contraction segment has been described with acid sensitive NCCP patients, but not with those with GERD [62]. Repetitive contraction of the smooth muscle segments may be seen in 'jackhammer esophagus', another hypercontractile motor disorder [63, 64] However, it is unknown whether these motor abnormalities can be seen in asymptomatic individuals, or if there is significant overlap with other esophageal disorders such as eosinophilic esophagitis and GERD. It is well known that perceptive symptoms such as chest pain may persist even when motor abnormalities are abolished pharmacologically [31]. While manometric abnormalities may play a role in symptom generation, they may not be solely responsible for symptoms, as manometric changes observed during clinical trials have not been influenced by treatment nor by clinical response [65]. Therefore, the true value of manometry, including HRM, in determining the cause of esophageal pain, and correlation of unexplained esophageal symptoms with motor disorders needs further study.

Other Tests

The balloon distention test has been used to demonstrate esophageal hypersensitivity in clinical studies but is infrequently used in practice [17]. Acid perfusion (Bernstein test) may reproduce chest pain symptoms in acid triggered chest pain, when compared to placebo saline infusion, but is another test used in research studies alone [60]. Additional techniques used to evaluate NCCP in research settings include esophageal evoked potentials (EEP) [66] and multimodal stimulation involving chemical, thermal, electrical and mechanical stimuli [67]. Psychological testing has been used to demonstrate symptom association with panic/anxiety disorders. EEPs are stimulus-specific voltage changes that occur after an esophageal stimulus and are used as neural measures of esophageal afferent pathway sensitivity [66]. Relatively noninvasive and inexpensive, EEPs are recorded with silver-silver chloride surface electrodes applied to the scalp and correspond to voltage changes that occur post esophageal stimulation. Profiles of optimal stimulation and recoding parameters such as latency and amplitude, relative to sensory and pain thresholds have been developed that can be used to identify changes in the esophageal afferent pathway or central sensitization [54, 66]. EEPs have thus far been used in the research setting to assess esophageal hypersensitivity and identify distinct phenotypic sub-groups within the NCCP population [66]; i.e. those individuals with NCCP as a consequence of sensitized afferents versus those with abnormal secondary processing of normal stimulation or hypervigilance [54].

Given the frequent psychological co-morbidity in patients with NCCP [60], psychological modeling has been investigated as tool to help discriminate between patients who present with chest pain [68]. In addition, the Hospital Anxiety and Depression scale (HADS) has been used to detect affective disorders in individuals with NCCP [69]. Psychological evaluation of NCCP patients with a positive HADS demonstrates that Type D personality or the tendency to experience emotional distress is associated with anxiety and depression symptoms and with panic disorder [70]. Difficulty identifying or verbalizing emotions (alexithymia) and anxiety sensitivity are also thought to contribute and increase symptom severity in NCCP [71]. Further, health care utilization was associated with an increase in alexithymia and anxiety sensitivity among men and women, respectively [71] Absence of CAD, atypical quality of chest pain, female sex, a younger age, and a high level of self reported anxiety have also been shown to correlate with higher levels of panic disorder among persons with chest pain [72]. Further evaluation by a psychologist or psychiatrist is warranted in those unresponsive to standard medical therapy, especially if there is suspicion of an underlying psychological comorbidity [60].

Management

In many instances, the diagnostic evaluation detailed above will identify a specific cause of NCCP; allowing for therapy tailored to the etiology. Additional therapies that have been

Table 3.2 Management options for esophageal chest pain

Treatment of GERD	Acid suppression (PPI, H2RA)
	Reflux reducing agents (baclofen, baclofen analogues)
	Antireflux surgery in select cases
Treatment of hypermotility	Smooth muscle relaxants (calcium channel blockers, nitroglycerin)
	Botulinum toxin injection into esophageal body or LES
	LES disruption in rare instances (pneumatic dilation, myotomy)
Treatment of hypersensitivity	Sensory neuromodulators (typically low dose antidepressants)
	Analgesics (gabapentin, pregabalin; narcotics not recommended)
	Theophylline
	Topical agents containing antacids, viscous lidocaine
	Acupuncture
	Hypnosis
	Other novel targets (prostaglandin E2 receptor, vanilloid receptor-1, and ASIC receptor modulation)
Treatment of psychiatric comorbidity	Contemporary antidepressants, antianxiety agents
	Cognitive and behavioral therapy
	Psychotherapy
Treatment of other esophageal conditions	Eosinophilic esophagitis (topical steroids, elimination diets)
	Infectious esophagitis (specific antiviral or antifungal agents as appropriate)

GERD gastroesophageal reflux disease, *PPI* proton pump inhibitor, *H2RA* histamine-2 receptor antagonist, *LES* lower esophageal sphincter

evaluated and are being currently investigated are also outlined below and in Table 3.2.

Antireflux Therapy

Acid suppression with a PPI is typically the first therapeutic measure initiated even prior to investigation for patients with NCCP. The benefits of short (1–2 weeks) and long term (6–8 weeks) PPI therapy for NCCP have been demonstrated in numerous clinical trials for individuals with and without pathologic reflux [18]. In randomized controlled trials, response to PPI therapy for NCCP ranges from 71 to 95 % [8, 18]. Acid suppression may also have value in patients with acid sensitivity despite absence of pathologic elevation in esophageal acid exposure. Notably, in one prospective randomized control trial, 39 % of NCCP patients without evidence of GERD by ambulatory 24 h pH study had a response to treatment with omeprazole [8]. Therefore, when there is response to PPI therapy, the medication can be continued, but tapered to the lowest effective dose that offers

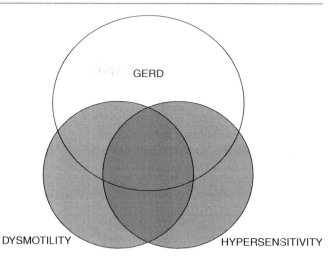

Fig. 3.4 Overlaps between gastroesophageal reflux disease, esophageal dysmotility and esophageal hypersensitivity in noncardiac chest pain. While each of these entities can exist independently, potential overlapping between two or all three can result in incomplete symptom resolution if only one entity is managed. Hypermotility is likely an epiphenomenon associated with hypersensitivity in many instances. Therefore, patients with esophageal hypersensitivity in the setting of gastroesophageal reflux disease, for instance, may have incomplete symptom relief unless both conditions are effectively treated

symptom relief. Other acid suppressive agents (e.g. H2 receptor antagonists, antacids) have not been studied in any detail in NCCP. As with typical GERD symptoms, non-pharmacologic measures (weight loss, avoidance of smoking and alcohol, avoiding lying down within 2–3 h of meals, sleeping with the head end of the bed elevated) may have value in conjunction with pharmacologic therapy.

Antireflux surgery is an option in patients with NCCP with well documented GERD, with abnormal esophageal acid exposure times. Patients with evidence of symptom-reflux correlation (especially positive SAP), and those who respond to PPI have a higher likelihood of symptom improvement after surgery.

Neuromodulators

If GERD is not evident or if it is thought to overlap with esophageal hypersensitivity (Fig. 3.4), the mainstay of therapy involves the use of pain modulators. Low dose antidepressants have been shown to be effective in reducing pain intensity and frequency of NCCP in patients with non GERD related NCCP [1, 73]. The tricyclic antidepressants (amitriptyline, nortriptyline, desipramine, imipramine) have been the most popular neuromodulators; trazodone and doxepin are related agents that share the benefits of tricyclic antidepressants. Tricyclic antidepressants may improve symptoms in as many as three quarters of patients with NCCP [73]. A long term follow-up study of NCCP successfully treated with low-dose tricyclic antidpressants has demonstrated that 75 % continue to use these medications effectively [73]. Treatment with non mood altering doses of trazodone (100–150 mg/day) resulted in a reduction in ratings of chest pain [65]. Side effects (drowsiness, urinary retention, dryness of the mouth, constipation, arrhythmias, priapism with trazodone) may be limiting, and may trigger decrease in dosage or switch to an alternate less potent agent [18].

Other classes of antidepressants have also been studied in NCCP. Treatment with long term selective serotonin reuptake inhibitors (SSRI) was effective in acid sensitivity, when citalopram 20 mg was administered daily for 6 months [74]. Sertraline started at 50 mg/day and titrated to a maximum of 200 mg/day was also found to be effective in improving NCCP in a randomized control trial [75].

Although data is limited in NCCP, other classes of neuromodulators may also have benefit in NCCP. GABA agonists such as gabapentin and pregabalin have been used in functional and neuropathic pain with benefit [76]. Topical agents including 2 % lidocaine may provide temporary relief of acute painful episodes [76].

Smooth Muscle Relaxants

Studies investigating treatment for nonspecific motility disorders have been mostly uncontrolled and limited by small sample size [18]. Smooth muscle relaxants that reduce esophageal contraction amplitude (sublingual nitroglycerine, phosphodiesterase-5 inhibitors, and calcium channel blockers) are frequently used, although their efficacy has not been conclusively demonstrated in controlled trials [18]. Unfortunately, decreasing contraction amplitude with muscle relaxants has not been demonstrated to reduce hyperalgesia inpatients with spastic motor disorders.

Botulinum Toxin Therapy

Botulinum toxin injected into the LES or the esophageal body has been studied in treatment of achalasia and other disorders with errors of LES relaxation. Botulinum toxin interferes with LES tone by irreversibly binding to cholinergic neurons. Although rarely used as a primary mode of therapy, botulinum injection is beneficial in achalasia patients as a bridge to more definitive therapy or as an alternative in those patients who are unable to undergo pneumatic dilation or Heller myotomy [77–79] There is some evidence to suggest that pain may improve if related to esophageal distension from incomplete bolus clearance. However, systematic improvement of esophageal pain has not been demonstrated [18]. In fact, a pain predominant presentation may be a marker of poor symptom relief with botulinum toxin injection in spastic motor disorders [78]. Response to botulinum toxin injection in individuals with incomplete LES relaxation lasted an average of 12.8 months; however, chest pain predominant symptoms, along with younger age and spastic features, predicted less durable and sub-optimal, short-term response (<6 mo) response [79]. In these individuals, consideration of alternative therapies such as neuromodulators, as discussed above, should be encouraged.

Other Approaches

Theophylline, an adenosine receptor antagonist, provided relief from functional chest pain in an open label trial [18]. After theophylline administration, patients with esophageal hypersensitivity to balloon distension increased their thresholds for discomfort and pain with graded balloon distention. Further, continuation of oral theophylline for 3 months resulted in sustained improvement in symptoms [80]. These findings have been subsequently confirmed in a randomized-placebo controlled trial [81]. However, the use of theophylline is limited by its side effect profile and toxicity. These studies demonstrate that the adenosine receptor could be a future potential target in the therapeutic armamentarium for NCCP [18, 82].

Prostaglandin E2 is a mediator of both central and peripheral sensitization and the prostaglandin E2 receptor (EP-1) has been implicated in esophageal acid-induced visceral hypersensitivity [53]. In a human model of esophageal secondary hyperalgesia, EP-1 antagonism was shown to diminish the pain threshold in the upper esophagus after acid infusion in the lower esophagus [53]. VR1 and ASIC receptor modulation are also potential novel targets for therapy in patients with hypersensitive esophagus [51].

Nonpharmacologic Approaches

Additional interventions including hypnotherapy, biofeedback, and transcutaneous nerve stimulation have been evaluated with some benefit, although additional studies are needed [18]. Finally, acupuncture can also be attempted in refractory situations [83, 84].

Prognosis

Identification of a specific etiology for NCCP improves the likelihood of symptom improvement, especially if NCCP is linked to GERD. Psychologic comorbidities, when prominent, predict continuing patient anxiety, distrust in the diagnosis, and continuing health care utilization.

References

1. Fass R, Malagon I, Schmulson M. Chest pain of esophageal origin. Curr Opin Gastroenterol. 2001;17(4):376–80.

2. Eslick GD, Fass R. Noncardiac chest pain: evaluation and treatment. Gastroenterol Clin North Am. 2003;32(2):531–52.

3. Lenfant C. Chest pain of cardiac and noncardiac origin. Metabolism. 2010;59 Suppl 1:S41–6.

4. Davies HA, Jones DB, Rhodes J, Newcombe RG. Angina-like esophageal pain: differentiation from cardiac pain by history. J Clin Gastroenterol. 1985;7(6):477–81.

5. Eslick GD. Chest pain: a historical perspective. Int J Cardiol. 2001; 77(1):5–11.

6. Fass R, Achem SR. Noncardiac chest pain: epidemiology, natural course and pathogenesis. J Neurogastroenterol Motil. 2011;17(2): 110–23.

7. Oranu AC, Vaezi MF. Noncardiac chest pain: gastroesophageal reflux disease. Med Clin North Am. 2010;94(2):233–42.

8. Pandak WM, Arezo S, Everett S, et al. Short course of omeprazole: a better first diagnostic approach to noncardiac chest pain than endoscopy, manometry, or 24-hour esophageal pH monitoring. J Clin Gastroenterol. 2002;35(4):307–14.

9. Kushnir VM, Sayuk GS, Gyawali CP. Abnormal GERD parameters on ambulatory pH monitoring predict therapeutic success in noncardiac chest pain. Am J Gastroenterol. 2010;105(5):1032–8.

10. Nasr I, Attaluri A, Hashmi S, Gregersen H, Rao SS. Investigation of esophageal sensation and biomechanical properties in functional chest pain. Neurogastroenterol Motil. 2010;22(5):520–6, e116

11. Locke 3rd GR, Talley NJ, Fett SL, Zinsmeister AR, Melton 3rd LJ. Prevalence and clinical spectrum of gastroesophageal reflux: a population-based study in Olmsted County, Minnesota. Gastroenterology. 1997;112(5):1448–56.

12. Eslick GD, Jones MP, Talley NJ. Non-cardiac chest pain: prevalence, risk factors, impact and consulting–a population-based study. Aliment Pharmacol Ther. 2003;17(9):1115–24.

13. Rey E, Rodriguez-Artalejo F, Herraiz MA, Alvarez-Sanchez A, Escudero M, Diaz-Rubio M. Atypical symptoms of gastro-esophageal reflux during pregnancy. Rev Esp Enferm Dig. 2011;103(3): 129–32.

14. Miwa H, Kondo T, Oshima T, Fukui H, Tomita T, Watari J. Esophageal sensation and esophageal hypersensitivity – overview from bench to bedside. J Neurogastroenterol Motil. 2010;16(4): 353–62.

15. Lasch H, Castell DO, Castell JA. Evidence for diminished visceral pain with aging: studies using graded intraesophageal balloon distension. Am J Physiol. 1997;272(1 Pt 1):G1–3.

16. Fass R, Pulliam G, Johnson C, Garewal HS, Sampliner RE. Symptom severity and oesophageal chemosensitivity to acid in older and young patients with gastro-oesophageal reflux. Age Ageing. 2000;29(2):125–30.

17. Fang J, Bjorkman D. A critical approach to noncardiac chest pain: pathophysiology, diagnosis, and treatment. Am J Gastroenterol. 2001;96(4):958–68.

18. Achem SR. Noncardiac chest pain-treatment approaches. Gastroenterol Clin North Am. 2008;37(4):859–78, ix.

19. Bautista J, Fullerton H, Briseno M, Cui H, Fass R. The effect of an empirical trial of high-dose lansoprazole on symptom response of patients with non-cardiac chest pain–a randomized, double-blind, placebo-controlled, crossover trial. Aliment Pharmacol Ther. 2004;19(10):1123–30.

20. Lee MM, Enns R. Narrow band imaging in gastroesophageal reflux disease and Barrett's esophagus. Can J Gastroenterol. 2009;23(2): 84–7.

21. Gawron AJ, Hirano I. Advances in diagnostic testing for gastroesophageal reflux disease. World J Gastroenterol. 2010;16(30): 3750–6.

22. Kushnir VM, Sayuk GS, Gyawali CP. The effect of antisecretory therapy and study duration on ambulatory esophageal pH monitoring. Dig Dis Sci. 2011;56(5):1412–19.

23. Prakash C, Clouse RE. Value of extended recording time with wireless pH monitoring in evaluating gastroesophageal reflux disease. Clin Gastroenterol Hepatol. 2005;3(4):329–34.

24. Prakash C, Clouse RE. Wireless pH monitoring in patients with non-cardiac chest pain. Am J Gastroenterol. 2006;101(3):446–52.

25. Richter JE, Barish CF, Castell DO. Abnormal sensory perception in patients with esophageal chest pain. Gastroenterology. 1986;91(4): 845–52.

26. Rao SS, Gregersen H, Hayek B, Summers RW, Christensen J. Unexplained chest pain: the hypersensitive, hyperreactive, and poorly compliant esophagus. Ann Intern Med. 1996;124(11): 950–8.

27. Borjesson M, Pilhall M, Eliasson T, Norssell H, Mannheimer C, Rolny P. Esophageal visceral pain sensitivity: effects of TENS and correlation with manometric findings. Dig Dis Sci. 1998;43(8):1621–8.

28. Winslow ER, Clouse RE, Desai KM, et al. Influence of spastic motor disorders of the esophageal body on outcomes from laparoscopic antireflux surgery. Surg Endosc. 2003;17(5):738–45.

29. Balaban DH, Yamamoto Y, Liu J, et al. Sustained esophageal contraction: a marker of esophageal chest pain identified by intraluminal ultrasonography. Gastroenterology. 1999;116(1):29–37.

30. Mujica VR, Mudipalli RS, Rao SS. Pathophysiology of chest pain in patients with nutcracker esophagus. Am J Gastroenterol. 2001; 96(5):1371–7.

31. Rao SS, Hayek B, Summers RW. Functional chest pain of esophageal origin: hyperalgesia or motor dysfunction. Am J Gastroenterol. 2001;96(9):2584–9.

32. Park H, Conklin JL. Neuromuscular control of esophageal peristalsis. Curr Gastroenterol Rep. 1999;1(3):186–97.

33. Yazaki E, Sifrim D. Anatomy and physiology of the esophageal body. Dis Esophagus. 2012;25(4):292–8.

34. Clouse RE, Carney RM. The psychological profile of non-cardiac chest pain patients. Eur J Gastroenterol Hepatol. 1995;7(12):1160–5.

35. Schey R, Dickman R, Parthasarathy S, et al. Sleep deprivation is hyperalgesic in patients with gastroesophageal reflux disease. Gastroenterology. 2007;133(6):1787–95.

36. Bradley LA, Richter JE, Pulliam TJ, et al. The relationship between stress and symptoms of gastroesophageal reflux: the influence of psychological factors. Am J Gastroenterol. 1993;88(1):11–9.

37. Sayuk GS, Elwing JE, Lustman PJ, Clouse RE. Predictors of premature antidepressant discontinuation in functional gastrointestinal disorders. Psychosom Med. 2007;69(2):173–81.

38. Prasad GA, Alexander JA, Schleck CD, et al. Epidemiology of eosinophilic esophagitis over three decades in Olmsted County, Minnesota. Clin Gastroenterol Hepatol. 2009;7(10):1055–61.

39. Croese J, Fairley SK, Masson JW, et al. Clinical and endoscopic features of eosinophilic esophagitis in adults. Gastrointest Endosc. 2003;58(4):516–22.

40. Noel RJ, Putnam PE, Rothenberg ME. Eosinophilic esophagitis. N Engl J Med. 2004;351(9):940–1.

41. Atkins D, Kramer R, Capocelli K, Lovell M, Furuta GT. Eosinophilic esophagitis: the newest esophageal inflammatory disease. Nat Rev Gastroenterol Hepatol. 2009;6(5):267–78.

42. Achem SR, Almansa C, Krishna M, et al. Eosinophilic oesophagitis in noncardiac chest pain: authors' reply. Aliment Pharmacol Ther. 2011;34(1):110.

43. Geagea A, Cellier C. Scope of drug-induced, infectious and allergic esophageal injury. Curr Opin Gastroenterol. 2008;24(4):496–501.

44. Clouse RE, Richter JE, Heading RC, Janssens J, Wilson JA. Functional esophageal disorders. Gut. 1999;45 Suppl 2:II31–6.

45. Mayer EA, Naliboff BD, Craig AD. Neuroimaging of the brain-gut axis: from basic understanding to treatment of functional GI disorders. Gastroenterology. 2006;131(6):1925–42.

46. Cannon 3rd RO. Causes of chest pain in patients with normal coronary angiograms: the eye of the beholder. Am J Cardiol. 1988; 62(4):306–8.

47. Cannon 3rd RO, Cattau Jr EL, Yakshe PN, et al. Coronary flow reserve, esophageal motility, and chest pain in patients with angiographically normal coronary arteries. Am J Med. 1990;88(3): 217–22.

48. Bennett J. ABC of the upper gastrointestinal tract. Oesophagus: Atypical chest pain and motility disorders. BMJ. 2001;323(7316): 791–4.

49. Zachariae R, Melchiorsen H, Frobert O, Bjerring P, Bagger JP. Experimental pain and psychologic status of patients with chest pain with normal coronary arteries or ischemic heart disease. Am Heart J. 2001;142(1):63–71.

50. Deval E, Gasull X, Noel J, et al. Acid-sensing ion channels (ASICs): pharmacology and implication in pain. Pharmacol Ther. 2010; 128(3):549–58.

51. Matthews PJ, Aziz Q, Facer P, Davis JB, Thompson DG, Anand P. Increased capsaicin receptor TRPV1 nerve fibres in the inflamed human oesophagus. Eur J Gastroenterol Hepatol. 2004;16(9):897–902.

52. Chauhan A, Petch MC, Schofield PM. Cardio-oesophageal reflex in humans as a mechanism for "linked angina". Eur Heart J. 1996;17(3): 407–13.

53. Sarkar S, Hobson AR, Hughes A, et al. The prostaglandin E2 receptor-1 (EP-1) mediates acid-induced visceral pain hypersensitivity in humans. Gastroenterology. 2003;124(1):18–25.

54. Hobson AR, Aziz Q. Brain processing of esophageal sensation in health and disease. Gastroenterol Clin North Am. 2004;33(1): 69–91.

55. Saito YA, Mitra N, Mayer EA. Genetic approaches to functional gastrointestinal disorders. Gastroenterology. 2010;138(4):1276–85.

56. Wang WH, Huang JQ, Zheng GF, et al. Is proton pump inhibitor testing an effective approach to diagnose gastroesophageal reflux disease in patients with noncardiac chest pain?: a meta-analysis. Arch Intern Med. 2005;165(11):1222–8.

57. Numans ME, Lau J, de Wit NJ, Bonis PA. Short-term treatment with proton-pump inhibitors as a test for gastroesophageal reflux disease: a meta-analysis of diagnostic test characteristics. Ann Intern Med. 2004;140(7):518–27.

58. Borzecki AM, Pedrosa MC, Prashker MJ. Should noncardiac chest pain be treated empirically? A cost-effectiveness analysis. Arch Intern Med. 2000;160(6):844–52.

59. Ofman JJ, Gralnek IM, Udani J, Fennerty MB, Fass R. The cost-effectiveness of the omeprazole test in patients with noncardiac chest pain. Am J Med. 1999;107(3):219–27.

60. Fass R, Achem SR. Noncardiac chest pain: diagnostic evaluation. Dis Esophagus. 2012;25(2):89–101.

61. Pandolfino JE, Ghosh SK, Rice J, Clarke JO, Kwiatek MA, Kahrilas PJ. Classifying esophageal motility by pressure topography characteristics: a study of 400 patients and 75 controls. Am J Gastroenterol. 2008;103(1):27–37.

62. Gyawali CP, Kushnir VM. High-resolution manometric characteristics help differentiate types of distal esophageal obstruction in patients with peristalsis. Neurogastroenterol Motil. 2011;23(6):502-e197.

63. Pandolfino JE, Roman S, Carlson D, et al. Distal esophageal spasm in high-resolution esophageal pressure topography: defining clinical phenotypes. Gastroenterology. 2011;141(2):469–75.

64. Roman S, Lin Z, Pandolfino JE, Kahrilas PJ. Distal contraction latency: a measure of propagation velocity optimized for esophageal pressure topography studies. Am J Gastroenterol. 2011;106(3): 443–51.

65. Clouse RE, Lustman PJ, Eckert TC, Ferney DM, Griffith LS. Low-dose trazodone for symptomatic patients with esophageal contraction

66. Hobson AR, Furlong PL, Sarkar S, et al. Neurophysiologic assessment of esophageal sensory processing in noncardiac chest pain. Gastroenterology. 2006;130(1):80–8.

67. Drewes AM, Reddy H, Pedersen J, Funch-Jensen P, Gregersen H, Arendt-Nielsen L. Multimodal pain stimulations in patients with grade B oesophagitis. Gut. 2006;55(7):926–32.

68. Serlie AW, Duivenvoorden HJ, Passchier J, ten Cate FJ, Deckers JW, Erdman RA. Empirical psychological modeling of chest pain: a comparative study. J Psychosom Res. 1996;40(6):625–35.

69. Kuijpers PM, Denollet J, Lousberg R, Wellens HJ, Crijns H, Honig A. Validity of the hospital anxiety and depression scale for use with patients with noncardiac chest pain. Psychosomatics. 2003;44(4): 329–35.

70. Kuijpers PM, Denollet J, Wellens HJ, Crijns HM, Honig A. Noncardiac chest pain in the emergency department: the role of cardiac history, anxiety or depression and Type D personality. Eur J Cardiovasc Prev Rehabil. 2007;14(2):273–9.

71. White KS, McDonnell CJ, Gervino EV. Alexithymia and anxiety sensitivity in patients with non-cardiac chest pain. J Behav Ther Exp Psychiatry. 2011;42(4):432–9.

72. Huffman JC, Pollack MH. Predicting panic disorder among patients with chest pain: an analysis of the literature. Psychosomatics. 2003;44(3):222–36.

73. Prakash C, Clouse RE. Long-term outcome from tricyclic antidepressant treatment of functional chest pain. Dig Dis Sci. 1999;44(12): 2373–9.

74. Viazis N, Keyoglou A, Kanellopoulos AK, et al. Selective serotonin reuptake inhibitors for the treatment of hypersensitive esophagus: a randomized, double-blind, placebo-controlled study. Am J Gastroenterol. 2012;107(11):1662–7.

75. Keefe FJ, Shelby RA, Somers TJ, et al. Effects of coping skills training and sertraline in patients with non-cardiac chest pain: a randomized controlled study. Pain. 2011;152(4):730–41.

76. Attal N, Cruccu G, Baron R, et al. EFNS guidelines on the pharmacological treatment of neuropathic pain: 2010 revision. Eur J Neurol. 2010;17(9):1113–e88.

77. Pasricha PJ, Ravich WJ, Hendrix TR, Sostre S, Jones B, Kalloo AN. Intrasphincteric botulinum toxin for the treatment of achalasia. N Engl J Med. 1995;332(12):774–8.

78. Porter RF, Gyawali CP. Botulinum toxin injection in dysphagia syndromes with preserved esophageal peristalsis and incomplete lower esophageal sphincter relaxation. Neurogastroenterol Motil. 2011;23(2):139–44. e127–8.

79. Prakash C, Freedland KE, Chan MF, Clouse RE. Botulinum toxin injections for achalasia symptoms can approximate the short term efficacy of a single pneumatic dilation: a survival analysis approach. Am J Gastroenterol. 1999;94(2):328–33.

80. Rao SS, Mudipalli RS, Mujica V, Utech CL, Zhao X, Conklin JL. An open-label trial of theophylline for functional chest pain. Dig Dis Sci. 2002;47(12):2763–8.

81. Rao SS, Mudipalli RS, Remes-Troche JM, Utech CL, Zimmerman B. Theophylline improves esophageal chest pain–a randomized, placebo-controlled study. Am J Gastroenterol. 2007;102(5): 930–8.

82. Achem SR. New frontiers for the treatment of noncardiac chest pain: the adenosine receptors. Am J Gastroenterol. 2007;102(5): 939–41.

83. Macpherson H, Dumville JC. Acupuncture as a potential treatment for non-cardiac chest pain – a survey. Acupunct Med. 2007;25(1–2):18–21.

84. Kim W, Jeong MH, Ahn YK. Acupuncture for chest pain. Heart. 2004;90(9):1062.

Rosanna Tavella and Guy D. Eslick

Abstract

Chest pain and normal coronary angiography is seen in up 30 % of patients undergoing the investigation. Despite its notable prevalence, the epidemiology of the condition remains poorly documented. Since the turn of the twentieth century, researchers have been baffled by "unmistakable" angina in the absence of coronary artery disease. Curiosity as to the cardiac aetiology of this chest pain became the focus of several key studies investigating the clinical and haemodynamic features of patients with normal coronary angiography. From these early findings, the cardinal features of three specific disorders associated with normal coronary angiography were established – Cardiac Syndrome X, Microvascular Angina and more recently, the Coronary Slow Flow Phenomenon. Although ambiguity in the literature exists, it is likely that an 'ischemic' mechanism for the chest pain in these patients is explained by coronary microvascular dysfunction. It also now understood that despite the absence of significant coronary artery disease, the outcomes of patients are not entirely favourable, with studies suggesting a frequent persistence of chest pain, and increased risk of cardiac events, particularly among women. This chapter will review the available epidemiological data on patients with chest pain and normal coronary angiography, and the clinical features and possible aetiological explanations for the specific coronary microvascular disorders.

Keywords

Normal coronary angiography • Prinzmetal's angina • Coronary heart disease • Myocardial ischemia • Cardiac syndrome X • Microvascular angina • Coronary slow flow pheonemon

R. Tavella, PhD, BSc (Hons)
Department of Medicine, The Queen Elizabeth
Hospital, The University of Adelaide,
28 Woodville Road, Woodville South,
Adelaide, SA 5011, Australia
e-mail: rosanna.tavella@adelaide.edu.au

G.D. Eslick, DrPH, PhD, FACE, FFPH (✉)
Department of Surgery, The Whiteley-Martin
Research Centre, The University of Sydney,
Sydney, NSW 2006, Australia
e-mail: guy.eslick@sydney.edu.au

Abbreviations

ACS	Acute coronary syndrome
CAD	Coronary artery disease
CHD	Coronary heart disease
CSFP	Coronary slow flow phenomenon
GUSTO	Global utilization of streptokinase and t-PA for occluded coronary arteries
MI	Myocardial infarction
NCA	Normal coronary angiography
TIMI	Thrombosis in myocardial infarction
WISE	Women's ischemia syndrome evaluation

J.C. Kaski et al. (eds.), *Chest Pain with Normal Coronary Arteries*,
DOI 10.1007/978-1-4471-4838-8_4, © Springer-Verlag London 2013

Definitions

Aetiology
The demonstration of the causes of disease.

Normal coronary angiography
Smooth epicardial coronary arteries or non-obstructive lesions (stenosis <50 %).

Prinzmetal's angina (variant angina)
Angina syndrome consisting of chest pain at rest resulting from myocardial ischemia caused by large vessel coronary vasospasm.

Prevalence
The number of people with the disorder at any give time.

Incidence
The number of new episodes of a disease over a period of time.

Coronary heart disease
A group of diseases involving the coronary vasculature resulting in myocardial ischemia due to impaired coronary blood flow. Coronary heart disease includes coronary atherosclerosis coronary artery spasm and/or coronary microvascular dysfunction.

Myocardial ischemia
A pathological state where myocardial tissues are compromised due to inadequate blood flow.

Cardiac syndrome X
Refers to patients with (i) exertional angina (ii) transistent ST segment depression during exercise stress testing, (iii) angiographically normal epicardial arteries and (iv) absence of other known cardiac causes of chest pain (such as coronary spasm, left ventricular hypertrophy or cardiomyopathy).

Microvascular angina
A group of patients with (i) chest pain (ii) abnormal coronary blood flow response to provocative vasomotor stimuli and (iii) angiographically normal epicardial arteries.

Coronary slow flow pheonemon
An angiographic finding characterised by delayed opacification of the distal vasculature despite the absence of obstructive epicardial coronary artery disease. The criteria that constitutes a diagnosis of the CSFP varies between researches. Some studies employ a Thrombolysis in Myocardial Infarction (TIMI) frame count of greater than 22 frames while others define the observation as three or more beats to opacify the vessel.

Epidemiological Considerations

Epidemiology, plainly translated from Greek, means "*the study of people*". Certainly, the term epidemiology refers to the study of diseases in populations, and specifically involves describing disease patterns, and identifying causes of diseases (aetiology), in order to provide data for disease prevention, evaluation, and management. Patients with chest pain and normal coronary angiography (NCA) are frequently labelled as having "syndrome X", reflecting the obscurity associated with this condition. This

chapter will endeavour to provide an overview of descriptions and causations regarding this condition, and specifically, on the recognised coronary microvascular disorders.

Considering the wide spectrum of information that epidemiology covers, this topic has not been comprehensively assessed in the setting of chest pain and NCA. In particular, prevalence and incidence data is not frequently available, in contrast to coronary heart disease (CHD) statistics, which are readily accessible. Although hospital-based cohort studies have investigated the characteristics and cardiac outcomes of patients with chest pain and NCA in general, epidemiological data on specific coronary microvascular disorders is sparse and is mostly limited to small research studies drawn from single centres. Other epidemiological data available are affected by the characterisation of study patients, for example, the extent to which they are investigated. Some studies have investigated the epidemiology of chest pain of "unknown" origin (i.e. populations drawn without information on coronary angiogram findings). Although the constitution of these samples is varied, useful information is still attainable. However, it should be noted that substantial ambiguity exists, and that further research is needed to gain a comprehensive epidemiologic picture of chest pain and NCA.

Defining Normal Coronary Angiography

Normal coronary angiography is defined as no visible disease, or non-obstructive atherosclerotic lesions (stenosis <50 % judged visually). The coronary angiogram provides a 'snapshot' of the coronary arterial lumen, and so when a coronary angiogram is labelled *normal*, in actual fact, it refers to a normal coronary lumen. A patient with NCA may have diffuse disease or localised lesions within the media of the coronary artery not identified by the coronary angiogram. Nonetheless, generally, the angiogram findings provide adequate information regarding the status of coronary blood flow. Thus, the coronary angiography has acquired predominance in the management of CHD. This has prompted focus on epicardial coronary artery disease (CAD), with little attention on the coronary microvessels. However it should be noted that the epicardial vessels usually contribute to less than 10 % of coronary vascular resistance, in contrast to the coronary microvessels, which are responsible for more than 70 % of the coronary resistance[1]. During the later half the twentieth century, as chest pain with NCA become recognised and investigated, important insights regarding the coronary microcirculation evolved.

Historical Evolution of 'Syndrome X'

Since the introduction of coronary angiography, it became clear that some patients with classic angina symptoms showed no evidence of significant coronary artery disease. This syndrome was first described in 1910 by William

Table 4.1 Landmark research findings in the study of 'syndrome X'

Study	N	Female	Patient features in addition to NCA
Likoff et al. 1967 [3]	15	15	Exertional chest pain, abnormal ECG at rest
Key findings: Normal hemodynamic response to exertion			
Arbogast and Bourassa 1973 [4]	10	6 F	Exertional chest pain
Key findings: ECG and transmyocardial lactate evidence of myocardial ischemia during atrial pacing			
Kemp 1973 [5]			
Introduced the term 'syndrome X' to define patients with exertional chest pain and NCA			
Opherk et al. 1981 [6]	21	6	Exertional chest pain, few ST segment changes
Key findings: All exhibited abnormal coronary blood flow response to vasomotor stimuli			
Some exhibited metabolic evidence of myocardial ischemia			
Cannon and Epstein 1988 [7]			
Introduced the term 'microvascular angina' to describe patients with evidence of dynamic microvascular dysfunction			
Tambe et al. 1972 [8]	6		Rest pain in one third, abnormal resting ECG
Key findings: Strikingly slow passage of contrast medium through the coronary arterial tree			
Beltrame et al. 2002 [9]			
Introduced the term 'coronary slow flow phenomenon' to describe delayed opacification of distal vasculature despite NCA			

Osler [2], who described this form of chest pain as "the chief difficultly" when diagnosing "true" angina pectoris. Coinciding with the more widespread use of coronary angiography, over the last 40 years research groups have investigated the mechanisms behind the "angina-like" chest pain. Several key studies have evolved the understanding of chest pain and NCA by examining the clinical and hemodynamic features of small groups of patients with chest pain and NCA. These studies generally indicated a reduced coronary flow reserve in patients however, not all patients demonstrated definitive evidence for myocardial ischemia. The clinical presentation of patients also differed, and although this may have just reflected the heterogeneous nature of the syndrome, it became clear that certain condition-specific characteristics had been recognised. Consequently, these conditions were labelled as *Syndrome X*, *Microvascular Angina*, and more recently, the *Coronary Slow Flow Phenomenon*. Detailed below are these key landmark findings in the studies of chest pain and NCA (Table 4.1)

Prevalence and Incidence Data

Chest Pain and Normal Coronary Angiography

Population based studies on the epidemiology and thus prevalence of chest pain and NCA are infrequent, and most studies are hospital-based. Furthermore, data on the incidence of the condition is rarely, if not ever, reported. Most likely, epidemiological statistics are not frequently available since there is lack of routine documentation of NCA in hospital administrative registries and thus a global lack of routine surveillance. Without true incidence data available to establish background population rates, it is difficult to assess the actual burden that

this condition imposes. Prevalence data is typically generated by tertiary referral centres, and with this, the resulting problems of referral bias, uncertainty of denominator population and the inclusion of only small samples should be noted.

Hospital-based studies have typically drawn populations from consecutive patients undergoing cardiac catheterization. These studies have generally revealed on average that around 20 % (range 6–31 %) of patients undergoing angiography for the investigation of angina-like chest pain show normal epicardial coronary arteries [10–13]. In regards to the specific coronary microvascular disorders, under-diagnosis and thus under-reporting make it difficult to evaluate the actual prevalence of these conditions. Furthermore, many studies in the medical literature consist of case reports and case series data by clinicians, with an emphasis on the clinical rather the epidemiological descriptions. These conditions will be further discussed later in the chapter.

Chest Pain of Unknown Origin

Other population-based studies that have investigated chest pain of "unknown" origin have not classified patients on the basis of coronary angiogram findings. These studies reflect the heterogeneous nature of the disorder since different criteria have been used to describe the condition. Thus, there is a considerable variation in prevalence of this chest pain. Geographically, there also seems to be variation in the epidemiology of the condition. As detailed in Fig. 4.1, low prevalence rates have been reported in Hong Kong [14] (14 %), whereas, a high prevalence has been reported in Australia (33 %) [15].

Although population based epidemiological studies have differed substantially in terms of methodology, it should be

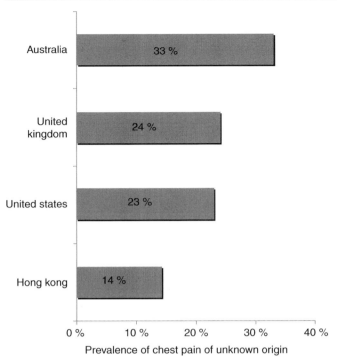

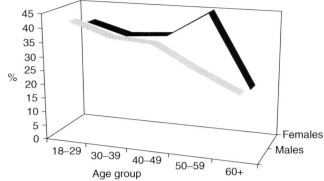

Fig. 4.2 Population prevalence of chest pain of unknown origin by age and gender (Reprinted from Eslick [18]. With permission from Elsevier)

Fig. 4.1 Geographical variation in the prevalence of chest pain of unknown origin. Note: Study definitions for chest pain of unknown origin. Australia [15]: (1) Chest pain that was not angina according to the rose angina questionnaire criteria, and (2) absence of ischemic heart disease as diagnosed by a doctor. Population, n=1,000, randomly selected from the community; United Kingdom [16]: (1) Non-exertional chest pain, (2) history of other prolonged chest severe pain and (3) absence of angina or myocardial infarction. Population, n=7,735, randomly selected from general practice, 100 % male; United States [17]: (1) Presence of chest pain but no self-reported history of cardiac disease. Population, n=1,511, selected randomly from the community; Hong Kong [14]: (1) Non exertional chest pain according to the Rose Angina Questionnaire and (2) absence of ischemic heart disease as diagnosed by a doctor. Population, n=2,209, selected randomly from the community

noted that most studies reveal several consistent findings: (a) a fairly significant prevalence of the condition (identified by coronary angiograms or other means); (b) decreasing prevalence with increasing age; and (c) an increased prevalence among females (Fig. 4.2 and Table 4.2).

Natural History of Chest Pain and Normal Coronary Angiography

Up to one third of patients undergoing coronary angiography for the evaluation of chest pain have NCA. However, the natural history of patients with significant CAD is well reported, the course of patients with NCA requires further exploration. In 1990, Chambers and Bass [23] presented a thorough review of the natural history of patients with chest pain and NCA, however, since then little prospective work

has been undertaken. Although long-term cohort studies have assessed mortality, the clinical characteristics and the results of non-invasive investigations also have not adequately described. This section will review current understanding of the clinical features and cardiac events associated with chest pain and NCA.

Clinical Features

Hospital based populations drawn from patients undergoing catheterisation typically show that the average age is in the late forties, similar to those with significant CAD. However, the proportion of males is smaller, with over 50 % commonly female. Of note, this female predominance is consistent irrespective of the definition used for sample inclusion. In contrast, the prevalence of cardiovascular risk factors has been shown to be similar to patients with CAD. One half of patients with NCA display ST or T wave changes and 25 % have ST segment depression on exercise. Interestingly, the episodes of ST segment depression are often indistinguishable from those observed in patients with CAD, particularly among Cardiac Syndrome X patients.

Chest Pain Characteristics

The description of chest pain is often simplified, particularly in research settings, as "typical" or "atypical" of cardiac origin. Due to the wide variation in interpretation and the subjective nature of descriptions, there is few objective data regarding chest pain characteristics in patients with NCA. Reports on the prevalence of pain that is typical of cardiac origin have ranged from 9 % [24] to over 50 % [25]. The uncertainty in the definitions, (i.e. how to define chest pain reproducible to exertion), contribute to the dissimilarities

Table 4.2 Prevalence of normal coronary angiography in females compared to males

	n/(%)		
	Females	Males	p
GUSTO [19]	343/1,768 (19 %)	394/4,638 (8 %)	<0.001
TIMI 18 [20]	95/555 (17 %)	99/1,091 (9 %)	<0.001
Unstable angina [19]	252/826 (31 %)	220/1,580 (14 %)	<0.001
TIMI IIIa [21]	30/113 (27 %)	27/278 (8 %)	<0.001
MI without ST-segment elevation [19]	41/450 (9 %)	55/1,299 (4 %)	0.001
MI with ST segment elevation [19]	50/492 (10 %)	119/1,759 (7 %)	0.02

Reprinted from Bugiardini, and Bairey Merz [22] with permission from American Medical Association
Abbreviations: GUSTO global utilization of streptokinase and t-PA for occluded coronary arteries, *TIMI* thrombosis in myocardial infarction, *MI* myocardial infarction

Fig. 4.3 Clinical characteristics of patients with normal coronary angiography. n=99, 78 females, all patients underwent cardiac catheterisation, exercise stress testing, ambulatory electrocardiography monitoring and echocardiography assessment. *ECG* electrocardiogram (Based on data from Kaski [26])

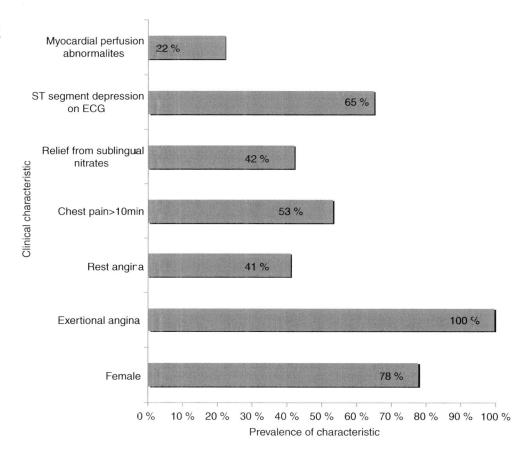

observed in these studies. Nonetheless, generally around 25 % of patients report pain typical of cardiac origin. It is thus well recognised that chest pain in patients with NCA includes many atypical features [10]. This is well described by Kaski [26], who discusses patients with NCA referred to a specialist pain clinic. The majority of patients reported pain that was typical for angina, but several atypical features were noted, including (1) chest pain at rest; (2) prolonged duration of pain; and (3) a poor response to sublingual nitrates (Fig. 4.3).

Cardiac Events

Long-term hospital-based cohort studies have demonstrated favourable prognosis in patients with chest pain and NCA, with the incidence of myocardial infarction or death almost 0 %. These studies show that myocardial infarction occurs in at most 1 % of patients, and death in 0.6 %, for follow-up periods for as long as 10 years [23]. Although these studies provide reassurance with regards to life expectancy, whether, a subgroup with poorer prognosis may have been

Table 4.3 Functional disability in patients with chest pain and NCA

Study	n	Hospital readmission (%)	Debilitated (%)	Physician consult (%)	Repeat coronary angiogram (%)	Ongoing cardiac medications (%)
Kemp, 1973 [10]	200	10				40
Bermiller, 1973 [31]	37				19	75
Day, 1976 [25]	45	5				25
Lavey, 1979 [32]	45	27	77	82	9	56
Ockene, 1980 [33]	57	15	51	71		25
Isner, 1981 [28]	121	18			3	64
Faxon, 1982 [34]	52	20	32			61
Bass, 1983 [35]	46		54			48
Papanicolaou, 1986 [13]	1,491	13	50			27
Lantinga, 1988 [36]	24		42	63		79

Reprinted from Chambers and Bass [23] with permission from Elsevier

concealed in these large cohorts remained largely unknown for several years.

In 2005, a systematic review revealed that the prognosis of patients with NCA may not be as benign as previously documented, in particular among those with unstable symptoms. This data indicate that patients with evidence of myocardial ischemia and NCA show a 2 % risk of death or myocardial infarction at 30-days follow-up [22]. Females, in particular, have a relatively poor prognosis compared to females with NCA and no evidence of myocardial ischemia. Data from the Women's Ischemic Syndrome Evaluation (WISE) [27] study indicate that this includes an increased risk for cardiovascular disease including sudden death, myocardial infarction and stroke.

Functional Outcomes

Morbidity poses a significant problem for patients with NCA, as many remain symptomatic. Around 75 % of patients continue to report persistent chest pain causing limitations in daily life activities. Episodes of persistent chest pain have been found to persist for as long as 4 years in many patients with NCA [28]. In addition, a significant proportion of individuals are unemployed due to the significant disability that persistent chest pain can cause. Thus, it is not surprising that patients continue to seek clinical advice, and this is despite some reports of anti-anginal treatment with multiple drug combinations [26, 29] (Table 4.3). Re-hospitalization for chest pain is also not infrequent, occurring in an estimated 20–50 % of patients. In addition, to the impact on individual functioning, the persistence of chest pain also increases the risk for adverse events. Among patients with NCA and coronary microvascular dysfunction, persistent chest pain is associated with increased risk of cardiovascular events, including myocardial infarction, heart failure and even sudden cardiac death [30].

Possible Causes of Chest Pain with Normal Coronary Angiography

Pain is a sensory and emotional experience, and since almost any structure in the chest may cause chest pain, there are many causes of chest pain to be considered in the setting of NCA. Accordingly, although patients with chest pain and NCA are often referred to as a distinct clinical entity, they undoubtedly represent a heterogeneous group of patients. When evaluating these patients, the first consideration is whether the pain is due to a cardiac but non-coronary aetiology, or secondly a non-cardiac cause (Table 4.4). In a small proportion of patients undergoing coronary angiography, *Printzmetal's* angina, identified by provocative spasm testing, may also explain chest pain in the absence of obstructive CAD.

Delineating between cardiac and non-cardiac causes of chest pain is difficult, as is differentiating between the various non-cardiac causes. Non-coronary conditions, such as cardiomyopathy or pericarditis, are usually obvious from patient history, clinical examination and routine cardiac investigations. It has been suggested that in up to 50 % of patients presenting with chest pain prompting medical attention, non-cardiac causes are implicated [38] and the chest pain may be attributed to a variety of disorders, including oesophageal abnormalities [39], musculoskeletal pain [40] and psychiatric disorders [41]. Several studies have attempted to determine the cause of chest pain, and a variety of approaches have been adopted to ascertain a diagnosis.

In Denmark, among patients who were admitted to hospital with acute chest pain but without myocardial infarction, a non-invasive screening programme revealed that 42 % of patients had gastroesophageal disease, 31 % showed ischemic heart disease, and 28 % has chest wall syndromes [42]. In a study by Husser et al. [43], 40 consecutive patients with NCA and no evidence of coronary spasm or syndrome X, underwent screening assessment for gastrointestinal, musculoskeletal and psychiatric causes of their chest pain. Although

Table 4.4 Differential diagnosis of chest pain and normal coronary angiography

Cardiac aetiologies	
Coronary causes	Variant angina (Prinzmetal angina)
	Syndrome X
	Microvascular angina
	Coronary slow flow phenomenon
Non-coronary causes	Pericarditis, myocarditis
	Cardiomyopathy
	Mitral valveprolapse
Non-cardiac aetiologies	
Respiratory system	Pneumothorax
	Pneumonia
	Pulmonary embolism
	Acute asthma
Gastrointestinal system	Oesophagitis, oesophageal spasm
	Gastroesophageal reflux
	Hiatus hernia
	Biliary colic, pancreatitis
Other causes	Chest wall syndromes, costochondritis (Tietze's syndrome)
	Psychogenic, panic attacks
	Munchausen syndrome

Based on data from Beltrame [37]

the sample size was small, 57 % had DSM-IV-R criteria for psychiatric disorders, 43 % had evidence of gastroesophageal reflux disease (i.e. responded to high dose proton pump inhibitor), and 16 % had evidence of a musculoskeletal cause on clinical examination (Fig. 4.4). It is important to note that regardless of the methodology employed to assess conditions, substantial overlap between the various causes is commonly reported.

Cardiac Causes

Although there are several potential causes of chest pain in patients with NCA who show no evidence of the above non-coronary causes of chest pain, the clinical suspicion has remained that these patients experience 'true' angina – the symptomatic manifestation of myocardial ischemia – in the absence of large vessel CAD. This is the group of patients frequently referred to as 'syndrome X'. A number of aetiological mechanisms for ischemia in the presence of normal coronary angiography have been proposed, including coronary small vessel disease [44].

Historically, these 'syndrome X' patients have been characterised by various approaches, as described in Section "Epidemiological Considerations". Specifically, these patients may be identified by the presence of 'ischemic' ST segment changes, abnormal coronary blood flow responses, or the delayed passage of contrast observed during coronary angiography (Table 4.1). Due to the limitations of coronary angiography,

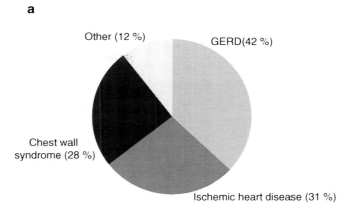

a

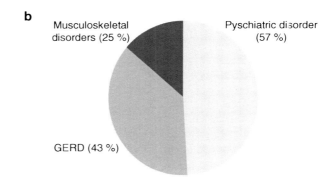

b

Fig. 4.4 (a) Differential diagnoses of patients admitted to hospital with acute chest pain n=204. Other includes perciarditis, pneuomina, pulmonary embolism, lung cancer, aortic aneurysm, aortic sterosis, and herpes zoster infection. *GERD* gastro-esophageal reflux disease (Adpated from Fruergaard et al. [42] with permission from Oxford University Press) (b) Differential diagnoses of patients with normal coronary angiography n=40. *GERD* gastroesophageal reflux disease (Based on data from Husser [43])

coronary microvascular disease is not readily recognised and diagnosed. Thus, the proportion of patients with chest pain patients and NCA that is explained by microvascular disease is undetermined.

In general, the prevalence of patients with typical exertional chest pain, positive exercise stress test and NCA is approximately 20 % of populations undergoing coronary angiography.

Adding to this, some studies suggest that coronary microvascular dysfunction is present in approximately 50 % of women with chest pain and NCA [45]. These patients tend to be younger, with the average age in the fifth decade of her life. It is suggested that the slow flow of dye in large coronary vessels is not an infrequent finding in patients during routine coronary angiography. In Europe, Mangieri et al. reports that this observation is prevalent in 7 % of patients with presenting with chest pain but normal coronary arteries [46]. Data from Australia report that the coronary slow flow phenomenon (CSFP) is seen in 1 % of the total diagnostic angiograms, based upon reports from the cardiologist performing the procedure [9]. More recent data from Australia suggest the CSFP is prevalent in 3 % of patients with NCA [47]. Australian findings are based upon the definition of three or more beats to opacity the left anterior descending artery.

Specific Coronary Microvascular Disorders

Abnormal vasomotor tone in the coronary microvessels has been implicated in patients with angina-like chest pain and NCA. Pathophysiologically, this may be explained by attenuated augmentation of coronary blood flow in response to increased myocardial oxygen demand [6, 48]. This may arise from excessive vasoconstriction or impaired compensatory vasodilatory mechanisms. In particular, endothelial dysfunction, with reduced bioavailability of endogenous nitric oxide and increased plasma levels of endothelin-1 (ET-1), may explain the abnormal behaviour of the coronary microvessels.

As outlined above, generally researchers have identified these patients on the basis of several approaches. However, coronary microvascular disorders are not readily identifiable and typically require specialised investigations that are usually performed in a research context. This section will discuss the clinical and pathophysiologic aspects of these coronary microvascular disorders.

Cardiac Syndrome X (Syndrome X)

Cardiac Syndrome X was first described in 1973 in relation to a landmark study by Arbogast and Bourassa [4]. This study evaluated transmyocardial lactate production in patients with exertional angina, a positive exercise test and either obstructive CAD (Group C) or no CAD (Group X) on angiography. Metabolic evidence of myocardial ischemia was demonstrated in both the Group C and X patients despite normal angiography in the later group. In the accompanying editorial by Kemp [10], he referred to the puzzling 'Group X' patients as 'Syndrome X'. This disorder should however, be distinguished from metabolic syndrome X, a condition characterised by insulin resistance, hyperglycaemia, hypertension, low high density lipoprotein cholesterol and raised triglycerides [49].

Syndrome X may be a generic term to describe patients with chest pain and NCA [50], and thus may be confused with large vessel coronary spasm. However, in its purest definition, Syndrome X patients are defined by certain characteristics (Table 4.5). In keeping with these specific criteria, the features of this disorder are summarised below. In regards to pathophysiology, numerous mechanisms have been proposed. Given the high prevalence of postmenopausal women in the Syndrome X population (approximately 70 %), estrogen deficiency has been suggested as a pathogenic agent acting via endothelium-dependent and endothelium-independent mechanisms. Despite the lack of metabolic evidence of myocardial ischemia in

Table 4.5 Cardiac syndrome X: definition and clinical features

Defining criteria for syndrome X

1. Exertional angina
2. ST segment depression on exercise testing
3. Absence of obstructive CAD on angiography
4. Absence of other cardiac disorders (coronary spasm, left ventricular hypertrophy, systemic hypertension, and valvular heart disease).

Clinical characteristics

Most often female

Typically present with prolonged episodes of exertional angina

Report significant disability due to on-going chest pain symptoms

Seldom experience myocardial infarction or cardiac death

Reported pathophysiological abnormalities

Myocardial ischemia

Abnormal coronary blood flow

Coronary microvascular abnormalities

Abnormal cardiac autonomic regulation

Endothelial dysfunction

Abnormal platelet aggregation

Abnormal pain perception

Metabolic and hormonal abnormalities

Systemic vascular abnormalities

Management

Beta-blockers effective in relieving chest pain

Nitrates are of limited benefit

Preliminary evidence showing a benefit with other therapies including:

    Enalapril, pravastatin, simvastatin, nicroandil

    Estradiol patches in women

    Impramine, transcutaneous nerve stimulators and spinal cord stimulation

Based on data from Beltrame [37]

patients, support for an 'ischemic hypothesis' includes the presence of surrogate markers of ischemia, such as sub-endocardial perfusion defects on magnetic resonance imaging [51] and reduction of high-energy phosphates on nuclear magnetic spectroscopy [52]. However, there is also evidence for a 'non-ischemic' hypothesis, including the demonstration of altered pain perception in these patients. It is likely that several pathways are important in the pathogenesis of Syndrome X.

Microvascular Angina

Initial studies characterising microvascular angina described patients with chest pain who showed reduced coronary blood flow response to atrial pacing despite the absence of large vessel disease [53]. A sub-group of patients also showed metabolic evidence of myocardial ischemia. Later studies documented similar results showing reduced vasodilator response to dipyridamole, and this supported an impaired dynamic response by the coronary resistance vessels to vasomotor stimuli [54]. Cannon and Epstein suggested that this

Table 4.6   Microvascular angina: clinical features

Clinical characteristics

Unlike syndrome X

   Infrequent display of ST changes on exercise stress testing

   Exertional angina is less commonly observed

Similar to syndrome X

   Females most often affected

   Resting left ventricular ejection fraction is usually normal

Among patients with left bundle branch block, a fall in ejection fraction with exercise is not uncommon

Pathophysiology

Few data in this condition, investigations have focused on:

   Generalised smooth muscle dysfunction

   Abnormal esophageal motility

   Bronchial hyper-responsiveness to methcholine

   Impaired forearm microvascular vasodilatory responses

   Increased sensitivity to cardiac and cutaneous nociceptive stimuli

   Association with anxiety states

Management

Calcium channel blockers may be of benefit

Few therapeutic studies undertaken

Table 4.7   Coronary slow flow phenomenon: clinical features

Clinical characteristics

Unlike Syndrome X and microvascular angina

   More often male

   Present with rest pain

Coronary angiography typically performed following ACS admission

Risk of subsequent MI is low

Re-admission for severe chest pain in one third of patients

Recurrent chest pain in 80 %

Pathophysiology

Involves abnormalities of the coronary microvasculature

   Elevated coronary vascular resistance

   Variable response to vasomotor stimuli

   Ventricular biopsy suggest presence of structural abnormalities

Management

Dipyrdiamole may be beneficial

Mibrefradil shown to be effective

Few therapeutic studies undertaken

Abbreviations: *ACS* acute coronary sydnrome, *MI* myocardial infarction

could be explained by abnormal prearterioal vasodilation in the coronary microcirculation, and referred to these patients as having 'microvascular angina'. This term is generally reserved for patients where coronary microvascular dysfunction is evidenced by abnormal coronary flow response to vasomotor stimuli. The clinical features of the disorder are summarised below (Table 4.6).

Coronary Slow Flow Phenomenon

The slow progression of dye down the coronary arteries in the absence of obstructive CAD was described by Tambe and colleagues in 1972 [8]. Recently, the Coronary Slow Flow Phenomenon (CSFP) has been defined as the angiographic observation of delayed opacification of epicardial vessels in patients with normal angiography [9]. Serial angiographic studies have demonstrated that the CSFP is persistent observation, although the severity of flow impairment may vary. Although in the literature there is disagreement on the diagnostic criteria to identify the presence of 'slow flow', the clinical features of the condition are well described (Table 4.7)

Conclusion

The understanding of patients with chest pain and normal coronary has undergone a prominent evolution since the condition was first noted at the turn of the twentieth century. Patients have historically been reassured the absence of heart disease and a benign prognosis. Contemporary data now call for a re-assessment of the outcomes associated with NCA. Many patients have persistence of symptoms, are re-hospitalised for chest pain and undergo a notable risk of cardiac events.

The specific disorders associated with NCA (Syndrome X, Microvascular Angina and CSFP) are well-characterised in terms of distinguishing clinical features. However, uncertainty still exists with regards to the diagnostic criteria and pathophysiological abnormalities. Since specialised investigations are typically required, there is a lack of large-scale epidemiological data leaving many questions unanswered. For example, the number of NCA patients with evidence of coronary microvascular disease and how this varies by country or region is not known, nor the number of new cases being diagnosed. Finally, uncertainty about the mechanisms of the symptoms makes management difficult. Due to a lack of epidemiological descriptions, the true impact of the NCA is likely underestimated.

Considering the functional impact that we are aware of, it is clear that additional large-scale clinical therapeutic studies are needed to determine effectiveness of treatment on chest pain symptoms. Future studies should also determine the value of less invasive methods of diagnosis. This may aid the feasibility of the fulfilling the need for urgent prospective epidemiological data.

References

1. Maseri A. The coronary circulation. In: Maseri A, editor. Ischemic heart disease. A rational basis for clinical practice and clinical research. New York: Churchill Livingstone; 1995. p. 71–104.
2. Osler W. The lumleian lectures on angina pectoris. Lancet. 1910; 175:697.

3. Likoff W, Segal BL, Kasparian H. Paradox of normal selective coronary arteriograms in patients considered to have unmistakable coronary heart disease. N Engl J Med. 1967;276(19):1063–6.

4. Arbogast R, Bourassa MG. Myocardial function during atrial pacing in patients with angina pectoris and normal coronary arteriograms. Comparison with patients having significant coronary artery disease. Am J Cardiol. 1973;32(3):257–63.

5. Kemp Jr HG. Left ventricular function in patients with the anginal syndrome and normal coronary arteriograms. Am J Cardiol. 1973;32(3):375–6.

6. Opherk D, et al. Reduced coronary dilatory capacity and ultrastructural changes of the myocardium in patients with angina pectoris but normal coronary arteriograms. Circulation. 1981;63(4):817–25.

7. Cannon 3rd RO, Epstein SE. "Microvascular angina" as a cause of chest pain with angiographically normal coronary arteries. Am J Cardiol. 1988;61(15):1338–43.

8. Tambe AA, et al. Angina pectoris and slow flow velocity of dye in coronary arteries – a new angiographic finding. Am Heart J. 1972;84(1):66–71.

9. Beltrame JF, Limaye SB, Horowitz JD. The coronary slow flow phenomenon – a new coronary microvascular disorder. Cardiology. 2002;97(4):197–202.

10. Kemp Jr HG, et al. The anginal syndrome associated with normal coronary arteriograms. Report of a six year experience. Am J Med. 1973;54(6):735–42.

11. Marchandise B, et al. Angiographic evaluation of the natural history of normal coronary arteries and mild coronary atherosclerosis. Am J Cardiol. 1978;41(2):216–20.

12. Pasternak RC, et al. Chest pain with angiographically insignificant coronary arterial obstruction. Clinical presentation and long-term follow-up. Am J Med. 1980;68(6):813–17.

13. Papanicolaou MN, et al. Prognostic implications of angiographically normal and insignificantly narrowed coronary arteries. Am J Cardiol. 1986;58(13):1181–7.

14. Wong WM, et al. Population based study of noncardiac chest pain in southern Chinese: prevalence, psychosocial factors and health care utilization. World J Gastroenterol. 2004;10(5):707–12.

15. Eslick GD, Jones MP, Talley NJ. Non-cardiac chest pain: prevalence, risk factors, impact and consulting–a population-based study. Aliment Pharmacol Ther. 2003;17(9):1115–24.

16. Lampe FC, et al. Chest pain on questionnaire and prediction of major ischaemic heart disease events in men. Eur Heart J. 1998;19(1):63–73.

17. Locke 3rd GR, et al. Prevalence and clinical spectrum of gastroesophageal reflux: a population-based study in Olmsted county, Minnesota. Gastroenterology. 1997;112(5):1448–56.

18. Eslick GD. Classification, natural history, epidemiology, and risk factors of noncardiac chest pain. Dis Mon. 2008;54(9):593–603.

19. Hochman JS, et al. Sex, clinical presentation, and outcome in patients with acute coronary syndromes. Global use of strategies to open occluded coronary arteries in acute coronary syndromes IIb investigators. N Engl J Med. 1999;341(4):226–32.

20. Glaser R, et al. Benefit of an early invasive management strategy in women with acute coronary syndromes. JAMA. 2002;288(24):3124–9.

21. Diver DJ, et al. Clinical and arteriographic characterization of patients with unstable angina without critical coronary arterial narrowing (from the TIMI-IIIA trial). Am J Cardiol. 1994;74(6):531–7.

22. Bugiardini R, Bairey Merz CN. Angina with "normal" coronary arteries: a changing philosophy. JAMA. 2005;293(4):477–84.

23. Chambers J, Bass C. Chest pain with normal coronary anatomy: a review of natural history and possible etiologic factors. Prog Cardiovasc Dis. 1990;33(3):161–84.

24. Waxler EB, Kimbiris D, Dreifus LS. The fate of women with normal coronary arteriograms and chest pain resembling angina pectoris. Am J Cardiol. 1971;28(1):25–32.

25. Day LJ, Sowton E. Clinical features and follow-up of patients with angina and normal coronary arteries. Lancet. 1976;2(7981):334–7.

26. Kaski JC, et al. Cardiac syndrome X: clinical characteristics and left ventricular function. Long-term follow-up study. J Am Coll Cardiol. 1995;25(4):807–14.

27. Johnson BD, et al. Prognosis in women with myocardial ischemia in the absence of obstructive coronary disease: results from the National Institutes of Health-National Heart, Lung, and Blood Institute-sponsored Women's Ischemia Syndrome Evaluation (WISE). Circulation. 2004;109(24):2993–9.

28. Isner JM, et al. Long-term clinical course of patients with normal coronary arteriography: follow-up study of 121 patients with normal or nearly normal coronary arteriograms. Am Heart J. 1981;102(4):645–53.

29. Chauhan A, et al. Clinical presentation and functional prognosis in syndrome X. Br Heart J. 1993;70(4):346–51.

30. Halcox JP, et al. Prognostic value of coronary vascular endothelial dysfunction. Circulation. 2002;106(6):653–8.

31. Bemiller CR, Pepine CJ, Rogers AK. Long-term observations in patients with angina and normal coronary arteriograms. Circulation. 1973;47(1):36–43.

32. Lavey EB, Winkle RA. Continuing disability of patients with chest pain and normal coronary arteriograms. J Chronic Dis. 1979;32(3):191–6.

33. Ockene IS, et al. Unexplained chest pain in patients with normal coronary arteriograms: a follow-up study of functional status. N Engl J Med. 1980;303(22):1249–52.

34. Faxon DP, et al. Therapeutic and economic value of a normal coronary angiogram. Am J Med. 1982;73(4):500–5.

35. Bass C, et al. Patients with angina with normal and near normal coronary arteries: clinical and psychosocial state 12 months after angiography. Br Med J (Clin Res Ed). 1983;287(6404):1505–8.

36. Lantinga LJ, et al. One-year psychosocial follow-up of patients with chest pain and angiographically normal coronary arteries. Am J Cardiol. 1988;62(4):209–13.

37. Beltrame J. Chest pain and normal angiography. In: Braunwald E, editor. Braunwald's heart disease e-dition. Philadelphia: Elsevier; 2006.

38. Mayou R, et al. Non-cardiac chest pain and benign palpitations in the cardiac clinic. Br Heart J. 1994;72(6):548–53.

39. Richter JE, Bradley LA, Castell DO. Esophageal chest pain: current controversies in pathogenesis, diagnosis, and therapy. Ann Intern Med. 1989;110(1):66–78.

40. Wise CM, Semble EL, Dalton CB. Musculoskeletal chest wall syndromes in patients with noncardiac chest pain: a study of 100 patients. Arch Phys Med Rehabil. 1992;73(2):147–9.

41. White KS. Assessment and treatment of psychological causes of chest pain. Med Clin North Am. 2010;94(2):291–318.

42. Fruergaard P, et al. The diagnoses of patients admitted with acute chest pain but without myocardial infarction. Eur Heart J. 1996;17(7):1028–34.

43. Husser D, et al. Evaluation of noncardiac chest pain: diagnostic approach, coping strategies and quality of life. Eur J Pain. 2006;10(1):51–5.

44. Bowling A. Measuring disease: a review of disease-specific quality of life measurment scales. Buckingham: Open University Press; 1995.

45. Reis SE, et al. Coronary microvascular dysfunction is highly prevalent in women with chest pain in the absence of coronary artery disease: results from the NHLBI WISE study. Am Heart J. 2001;141(5):735–41.

46. Mangieri E, et al. Slow coronary flow: clinical and histopathological features in patients with otherwise normal epicardial coronary arteries. Cathet Cardiovasc Diagn. 1996;37(4):375–81.

47. Jesuthasan L, Beltrame J, Marwick TH. Prevalence of coronary slow flow in patients undergoing coronary angiogram in a large teaching hospital. Heart Lung Circ. 2009;18(3):S121.

48. Camici PG, et al. Coronary hemodynamics and myocardial metabolism in patients with syndrome X: response to pacing stress. J Am Coll Cardiol. 1991;17(7):1461–70.

49. Grundy SM, et al. Definition of metabolic syndrome: report of the National Heart, Lung, and Blood Institute/American Heart Association conference on scientific issues related to definition. Circulation. 2004;109(3):433–8.

50. Maseri A. Syndrome X and microvascular angina. In: Maseri A, editor. Ischemic heart disease. A rational basis for clinical practice and clinical research. New York: Churchill Livingstone; 1995. p. 507–32.

51. Panting JR, et al. Abnormal subendocardial perfusion in cardiac syndrome X detected by cardiovascular magnetic resonance imaging. N Engl J Med. 2002;346(25):1948–53.

52. Buchthal SD, et al. Abnormal myocardial phosphorus-31 nuclear magnetic resonance spectroscopy in women with chest pain but normal coronary angiograms. N Engl J Med. 2000;342(12): 829–35.

53. Cannon 3rd RO, et al. Angina caused by reduced vasodilator reserve of the small coronary arteries. J Am Coll Cardiol. 1983;1(6): 1359–73.

54. Beltrame JF, et al. The prevalence of weekly angina among patients with chronic stable angina in primary care practices: The Coronary Artery Disease in General Practice (CADENCE) Study. Arch Intern Med. 2009;169(16):1491–9.